FACULTY DEVELOPMENT WORKBOOK

TEACHER TRAINING BOOT CAMP

FACULTY DEVELOPMENT WORKBOOK

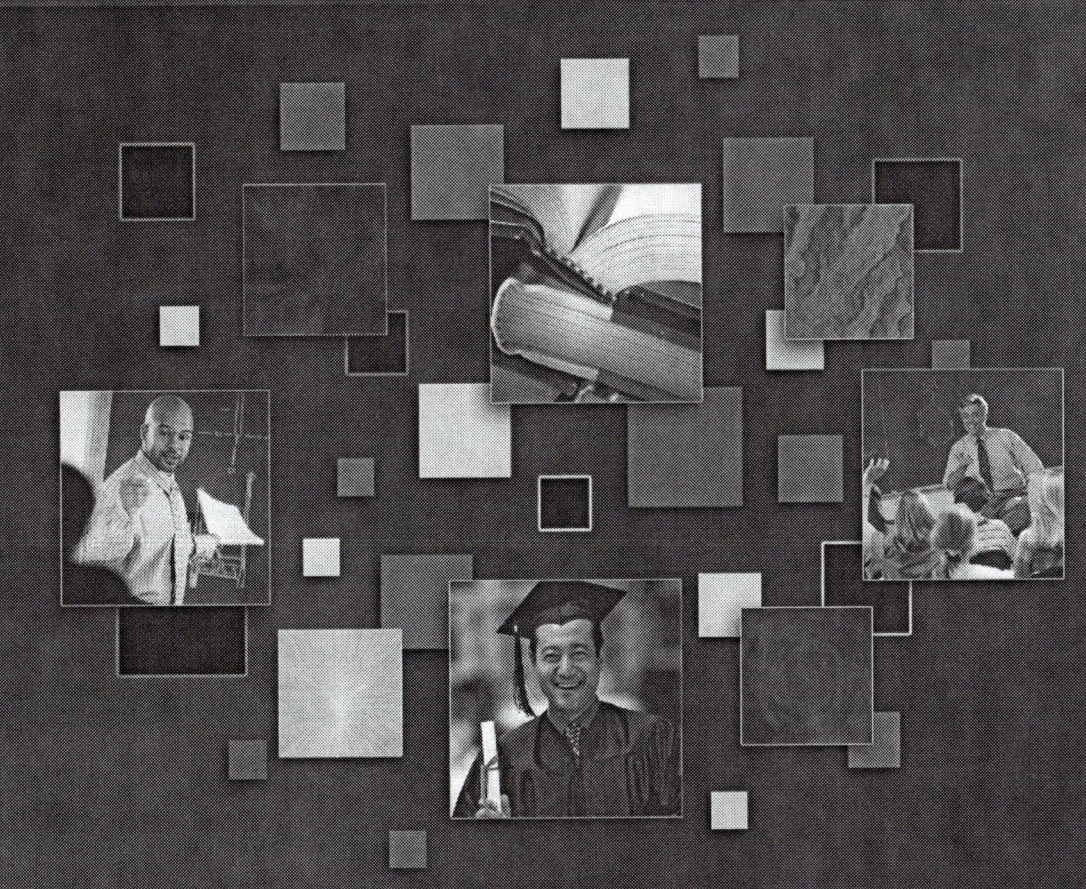

TEACHER TRAINING
BOOT CAMP

Amy Solomon, MS, OTR

Quantum Integrations

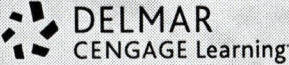

DELMAR
CENGAGE Learning™

Australia • Brazil • Japan • Korea • Mexico • Singapore • Spain • United Kingdom • United States

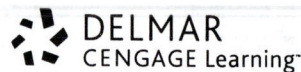

Faculty Development Workbook: Teacher Training Boot Camp
Amy Solomon

Vice President, Career Education SBU: Dawn Gerrain

Acquisitions Editor: Martine Edwards

Managing Editor: Robert L. Serenka, Jr.

Developmental Editor: Jennifer Anderson

Editorial Assistant: Falon Ferraro

Director of Production: Wendy A. Troeger

Production Manager: J.P. Henkel

Content Project Manager: Amber Leith

Director of Marketing: Wendy E. Mapstone

Channel Manager: Gerard McAvey

Compositor: Interactive Composition Corporation

> For product information and technology assistance, contact us at
> **Cengage Learning Customer & Sales Support, 1-800-354-9706**
> For permission to use material from this text or product,
> submit all requests online at **cengage.com/permissions**
> Further permissions questions can be emailed to
> **permissionrequest@cengage.com**

ISBN-13: 978-1-4180-4800-6

ISBN-10: 1-4180-4800-3

Delmar
Executive Woods
5 Maxwell Drive
Clifton Park, NY 12065
USA

Cengage Learning is a leading provider of customized learning solutions with office locations around the globe, including Singapore, the United Kingdom, Australia, Mexico, Brazil, and Japan. Locate your local office at:
international.cengage.com/region

Cengage Learning products are represented in Canada by Nelson ? Education, Ltd.

For your lifelong learning solutions, visit **delmar.cengage.com**

Visit our corporate website at **www.cengage.com**

Printed in the United States of America
2 3 4 5 6   14 13 12 11 10

ED176

CONTENTS

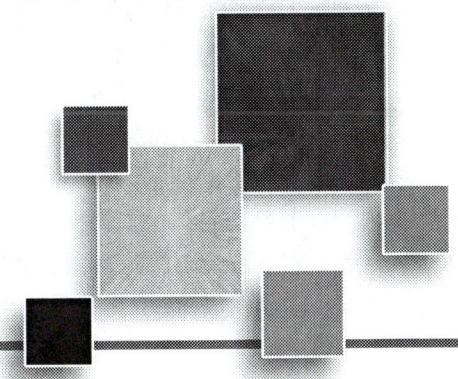

SECTION 2   Preparing to Teach and the First Days of Class   **43**

SECTION 3   The Day-to-Day Classroom Environment   **69**

SECTION 4   Grading and Assessment   105

INTRODUCTION

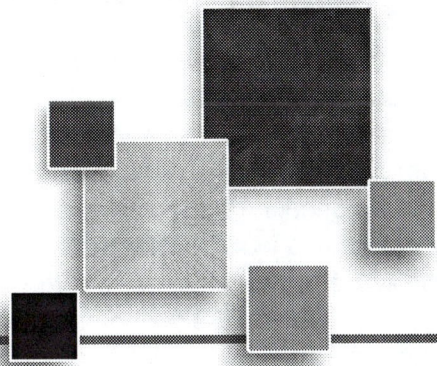

DELMAR'S FACULTY DEVELOPMENT SERIES

Delmar's Faculty Development Series consists of a collection of online courses covering a wide range of topics relevant to contemporary education and the development of quality teaching practices. In addition to course content, the online courses offer added value through features that support practical application of the material, including reflection questions, activities, ideas for classroom activities and assignments, professional portfolio development, and a tool for setting and tracking professional development goals.

HOW TO USE THIS WORKBOOK

The Faculty Development Workbook is offered as a guide and supplement to the main online course. Each workbook is customized to the content of its corresponding online course and is intended to customize the online content to individual needs. Because access to the online component has time constraints, completing each module's corresponding workbook provides a permanent reference for material once access to the online course has expired. Completing the workbook will provide you with a guide that includes a "refresher" course of material covered, ideas for development of your curriculum and courses over time, and methods for continued development of your teaching skills.

Workbook Components and Their Applications

Each workbook contains elements that correspond to the items found in its corresponding online course. Before using the workbook, take the time to understand how each element can be used to support you in completing the online course and to develop a resource for future reference.

Main Headings

Each of the main headings found in the online course is represented in the workbook. Space is provided for you to make notes of important concepts, ideas, and most importantly, to customize the information to your own needs. These notes will be your main resource after your access time to the online course has expired, so using this feature to its maximum potential will be of great benefit in the future.

Take It to the Classroom Activities

Take It to the Classroom activities are learning activities for you to use in your classroom with students. They are designed to provide you with specific activities that you can use immediately in the classroom and to help you apply the concepts of the online course. Some activities may be more appropriate for your group of students than others, and you are encouraged to select activities that fit your needs. One benefit of having the completed workbook is that you will be able to refer back to and select different activities as you teach classes with various needs each term. Space for planning each activity is provided. The online component provides the background needed to meet the goal of each activity.

Learning Activities

The Learning Activities provided at the conclusion of each section are capstone activities intended to synthesize the concepts from the section and provide an opportunity to apply them in practical situations. Activities include individual, group, and online formats, and the background needed to meet the goal of each activity is provided in the online component.

Activity Files

Throughout the online courses, activities are provided to illustrate main concepts, support the development of teaching skills, and conduct assessments of goal achievement. Completion of the Activity Files supports achievement of section learning objectives. The goals of these activities are also supported by online course content, and their successful completion provides the foundation for the capstone learning activities at the end of each section. Activity sheets and instructions are provided in both the online course and in the workbook.

Learning Objectives Revisited

Learning objectives are listed at the beginning of each section. Mastery of the online content and completion of the reflection questions and activities contribute to the achievement of the objectives. Learning Objectives Revisited provides you with a tool for assessing your own learning and setting goals for future development in areas covered in the section. The completed workbook will be a valuable resource to you in achieving this goal after your access to the online course has expired.

Instructor Improvement Plan

The Instructor Improvement Plan is designed as a long-term professional development tool. It provides a mechanism for setting individual goals in areas important to your professional development. The tool provides a means for recording goals, time frames, and methods for completion, as well as the opportunity to modify goals over time. One Instructor Improvement Plan form is provided for each module. You are encouraged to make a copy for each section and set individual goals for each section. You may wish to use this tool as part of your school's professional development and faculty assessment program.

Professional Development Portfolio

The Professional Development Portfolio is a collection of learning activities that you have completed and that serve as documentation of your professional development. Portfolios can be used as records of your professional development or to document your achievements to supervisors or other professional colleagues. Each module provides a guide for creating a Professional Development Portfolio based on module content. You are encouraged to modify this guide as necessary to support your interests and needs.

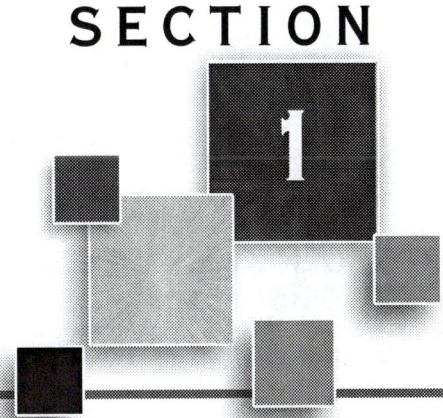

SECTION 1

AN OVERVIEW OF INSTRUCTOR RESPONSIBILITIES AND LEARNING THEORY

LEARNING OBJECTIVES

Upon successful completion of Section 1, the instructor will have achieved the following objectives. Check off each of the objectives as you have mastered it. You will have the opportunity to assess your performance on each objective at the end of Section 1.

1. The instructor will identify several responsibilities in teaching adults and explain the importance of these responsibilities to the success of the student and the institution.
2. The instructor will be able to describe general characteristics of adult learners and explain specific ways that knowledge of these characteristics can be used to increase the opportunity for learning in classrooms and training facilities.
3. The instructor will be able to describe specific learning and instruction theories and identify specific ways that he or she can use the information to enhance teaching strategies.

INTRODUCTORY QUESTIONS

- What are your responsibilities as an instructor of a course or workshop?
- What are some characteristics of your adult students? (Describe several specific characteristics of your students.)
- What learning or instructional theories do you know?
- Why is it important to understand how adults learn?

OVERVIEW

Section 1 briefly identifies several responsibilities of the instructor of adult learners in academic or training situations. It focuses on basic principles important to instructors of adults in an academic or training environment. General guidelines are suggested for the first-time instructor (and they apply to seasoned instructors as well). A brief overview of adult learner characteristics is presented, including specific ways instructors can apply this information in their classrooms. Section 1 also discusses several learning and instructional theories that can significantly improve learning opportunities for the adult student. "Take It to the Classroom" activities provide suggestions for actively applying concepts to your classes.

SUGGESTED GENERAL GUIDELINES: RESPONSIBILITIES OF INSTRUCTORS

Based on the information in the online module, summarize each of the following responsibilities of a college instructor.

Provide High-Quality Instruction

Complete Institutional Administrative Tasks

Accurately and Equitably Evaluate and Grade Students

Retain Students in Classes and in the Institution

Keep Current in the Field and Grow as a Teacher

Be sure to record your answers to these questions in the space provided and file them in the appropriate section of your Professional Development Portfolio.

- In addition to the above general responsibilities, what specific responsibilities do you have related to teaching in your institution? Write these down in a checklist format.

_____

_____

_____

_____

_____

- In what specific areas on your list might you need to improve?

_____

_____

_____

_____

_____

- What specific strategies are you going to use to help retain students in your class?

_____

_____

_____

_____

_____

- What specific steps do you take to keep current in your field and continuously grow as a teacher? What additional steps could you take?

_____

_____

_____

_____

_____

DEVELOPING UNDERSTANDING AND EMPATHY FOR STUDENTS

Summarize each of the bulleted points from the online module. Note areas in which you would like to develop your knowledge and skills.

■ ■ ■ DIVERSITY CONSIDERATIONS ■ ■ ■

Part of understanding students and developing empathy is respecting diversity in all of its forms. A student's cultural background can influence the manner in which he or she views instructors. For example, students from some cultures may view the instructor as an authority figure and be reluctant to ask questions or express a divergent opinion. Be aware of cultural and other types of diversity in your students and be aware of their impact on class dynamics.

DIVERSITY REFLECTIONS

• What other diversity issues might you encounter in the classroom?

_____

_____

_____

_____

_____

• How would you respond to these situations?

_____

_____

_____

_____

_____

REFLECTION QUESTIONS

Be sure to record your answers to these questions in the space provided and file them in the appropriate section of your Professional Development Portfolio.

- What is your impression of the students you teach or will be teaching? (Describe your students in detail.) Why do you perceive them as you do?

_____

_____

_____

_____

_____

- If you decided to go back to school, starting this term, what obstacles would you face in your own life? (Write down as many obstacles as you can identify.) Which of these might also apply to your students?

_____

_____

_____

_____

_____

- How would you reduce or overcome each of these limitations?

_____

_____

_____

_____

_____

ADULT LEARNERS IN A NUTSHELL

Note the importance of understanding the unique characteristics of adult learners.

Adult Learners Have Many Life Experiences

Record the importance of adult learners' life experiences and describe an effective interactional style on the part of the instructor.

```



```

GENERAL STRATEGIES FOR INCORPORATING STUDENTS' LIFE EXPERIENCES

Note strategies for recognizing and honoring students' life experiences. In addition to those suggested in the module, add your own ideas.

```



```

Adult Learners Have Past Educational Experiences

Comment on the effects that past educational experiences can have on adult learners.

```



```

GENERAL STRATEGIES FOR ACKNOWLEDGING STUDENTS' PAST EDUCATIONAL EXPERIENCES

Note strategies for taking into consideration students' past educational experiences. In addition to those suggested in the module, add your own ideas.

```



```

Each Learner Has Different Learning Abilities, Thinking Mechanisms, and Cognitive Processing Styles

Record your understanding of various learning and cognitive styles. Note topics about which you would like to learn more.

GENERAL STRATEGIES FOR SUPPORTING DIFFERENT LEARNING AND COGNITIVE STYLES

Note strategies for supporting students' various learning and cognitive styles. In addition to those suggested in the module, add your own ideas.

Adults Have Responsibilities That Must Often Come Before Their Education

Note the numerous responsibilities that adult learners have in addition to school. Comment on the approach the instructor can use to support adult learners' success.

GENERAL STRATEGIES FOR RESPECTING ADULTS' RESPONSIBILITIES

Note strategies for supporting adult learners' numerous responsibilities. In addition to those suggested in the module, add your own ideas.

■ ■ ■ DIVERSITY CONSIDERATIONS ■ ■ ■

An example of cultural diversity that can affect a student's attendance is the student from a culture where it is considered a primary responsibility to care for an older relative who is ill. A student from a culture such as this will probably prioritize cultural responsibility over school. A flexible policy will allow for consideration of this cultural priority.

DIVERSITY REFLECTIONS

- How can classroom policy be flexible and equitable at the same time?

_____

_____

_____

_____

_____

Adult Learners Are Goal-Oriented

Note common reasons that adults return to school.

GENERAL STRATEGIES FOR SUPPORTING STUDENTS' GOALS

Note strategies for supporting students' individual goals. In addition to those suggested in the module, add your own ideas.

Adults Have Made Significant Financial Investments in Their Education

Make a note of the financial significance of school for most adult learners.

GENERAL STRATEGIES FOR SUPPORTING STUDENTS' FINANCIAL INVESTMENTS

Note strategies for adding value to students' financial investment. In addition to those suggested in the module, add your own ideas.

Adults Value Autonomy and Self-Direction

Summarize typical adult learners' attitudes toward autonomy and their investment in their education.

GENERAL STRATEGIES FOR ENCOURAGING AUTONOMY

Note strategies for encouraging and supporting autonomy in your adult students. In addition to those suggested in the module, add your own ideas.

Adults Seek Relevant and Practical Information

Comment on the importance of relevant information to adult learners.

GENERAL STRATEGIES FOR MAKING INFORMATION RELEVANT AND PRACTICAL

Record strategies for making information relevant and practical. In addition to those suggested in the module, add your own ideas.

Adults Respond Best to Certain Teaching Methods

Summarize teaching methods that are most appropriate for adults and state why these approaches are most effective.

GENERAL STRATEGIES FOR USING EFFECTIVE LEARNING METHODS

Note strategies for incorporating effective teaching methods into your classroom. In addition to those suggested in the module, add your own ideas.

REFLECTION QUESTIONS

Be sure to record your answers to these questions in the space provided and file them in the appropriate section of your Professional Development Portfolio.

- What additional applications can you think of to meet the needs of adult learners? (Try to identify at least three additional specific applications for each characteristic in the list above.)

_____

_____

_____

_____

_____

- Which ones sound like good ideas for your own classes?

_____

_____

_____

_____

_____

_____

TAKE IT TO THE CLASSROOM ACTIVITIES

Take It to the Classroom activities are designed to support you in applying the module's concepts to the classroom. Course objectives will be met most effectively and learning will be most beneficial if the activities are completed in conjunction with the material found in the online course.

Student Autobiographies

Ask students to write their autobiographies from the perspective of how their life events have influenced their perspectives on school and learning. Suggest that they consider their educational, professional, and general life experiences. Share the results in class if time permits and if students are willing to share. Other options include collecting the papers and using them confidentially with each student or allowing students to keep their papers for their own use and insight. Be sure to explain to students the purpose of this activity and the goals you wish to achieve by using it. Student Autobiographies may be useful in subsequent activities in this section.

Notes for Planning This Activity:

Study Guides

Help students (especially those returning to school after an extended time) practice effective study skills for your class. On assignment sheets, include study tips that are relevant to each assignment. For example, an effective recommendation for studying anatomy and physiology is to draw and label the body parts. When creating study guides, consider methods that best support the material and that reflect a variety of learning styles.

Notes for Planning This Activity:

Learning Style Inventories

Conduct an Internet search using "Learning Style Inventory" as your search term. Ask students to take one that you recommend (or they can choose their own) and ask them to devise ways they can adapt their studying to match their learning style.

Notes for Planning This Activity:

What Makes Your Perspective?

Help students to understand their perspectives and to develop reflective thinking skills by asking them to evaluate the experiences, viewpoints, and other factors that influence their perspectives on a particular topic. Ask students to discuss their conclusions in small groups, pairs, or in brief written summaries. A class discussion will help students understand the diverse influences that affect learning. Emphasize to students that they need share only what they are comfortable sharing.

Notes for Planning This Activity:

Classroom Policy Input

Review classroom policies with students at the beginning of the term and seek their input on the flexibility and fairness of those policies. Of course, you have the final say and are responsible for seeing that the policies are in compliance with school policy and regulatory guidelines. Within these parameters, students are typically fair, yet maintain high standards. Remember that most people are highly invested in what they have helped to develop.

Notes for Planning This Activity:

Goals Journal

Ask students to clearly identify their professional goals and to keep semi-weekly journals that explore how course content applies to and supports their goals. Students may wish to refer to their autobiographies (if they have written them) as well as incorporate other reflective thinking activities into their goals journal. With the students' permission, these journals may be useful in student coaching and advising.

Notes for Planning This Activity:

The "Real" World

Bring as many elements of the actual professional workplace as possible into your classroom. Depending on the content and subject of your course, different techniques such as field trips, guest speakers, or panel discussions may be most appropriate. Evaluate your course for the most effective method. During these activities, emphasize the relationship of your course material to the workplace. Engaging outside professionals in applying the concepts contributes to helping students make the connection between education and the professional role.

Notes for Planning This Activity:

A FEW *DON'TS* FOR INSTRUCTORS OF ADULTS

Note strategies to avoid when teaching adult learners.

SELECTED EDUCATIONAL THEORIES FOR THE ADULT LEARNER

List the resources provided for additional information regarding educational theory that is appropriate for the adult learner.

Learning Styles

Note the important concepts of learning styles. Sketch the diagram from the online module for your future reference.

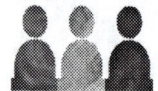

■ ■ ■ DIVERSITY CONSIDERATIONS ■ ■ ■

Although we do not typically think of learning styles as an element of diversity, they indeed contribute to variety in the classroom. Begin to view different learning styles and thought processes as another element of diversity and individuality among your students.

DIVERSITY REFLECTIONS

- What situations can you think of (in class or other circumstances) where differences in learning style needed consideration? What approach did you take?

_____

_____

_____

_____

_____

GENERAL STRATEGIES FOR VISUAL LEARNERS

Describe the visual learner. List effective strategies to use in class to support visual learners.

GENERAL STRATEGIES FOR DEVELOPING VISUAL LEARNING SKILLS

Record methods for encouraging all students to develop their visual learning skills.

GENERAL STRATEGIES FOR AUDITORY LEARNERS

Describe the auditory learner. List teaching strategies that effectively support the auditory learner.

GENERAL STRATEGIES FOR DEVELOPING AUDITORY LEARNING SKILLS

List methods that can be used to support all students in developing their auditory learning skills.

GENERAL STRATEGIES FOR KINESTHETIC LEARNERS

Describe the kinesthetic learner. List teaching strategies that are effective when teaching the kinesthetic learner.

GENERAL STRATEGIES FOR DEVELOPING KINESTHETIC LEARNING SKILLS

Record methods you can use to support all students in developing their kinesthetic learning skills.

See the *Addressing Different Learning Styles Checklist* at the end of this section.

REFLECTION QUESTIONS

Be sure to record your answers to these questions in the space provided and file them in the appropriate section of your Professional Development Portfolio.

- What is your personal learning style?

_____

_____

_____

_____

_____

- How do you think your personal learning style affects your teaching style?

_____

_____

_____

_____

_____

- What learning style do you think is least addressed by your teaching style? Best addressed?

_____

_____

_____

_____

_____

Bloom's Taxonomy

Summarize each of the following components of Bloom's taxonomy and draw the diagram that represents the levels of the cognitive domain. Provide an example of a classroom activity that represents each level.

Knowledge

Comprehension

Application

Analysis

Synthesis

Evaluation

See the *Bloom's Taxonomy Word List* at the end of this section.

REFLECTION QUESTIONS

Be sure to record your answers to these questions in the space provided and file them in the appropriate section of your Professional Development Portfolio.

- Review the learning objectives for your course. To what level of Bloom's taxonomy does each objective apply?

_____

_____

_____

_____

_____

The Cognitive Apprenticeship Model

Summarize each of the steps of the Cognitive Apprenticeship Model listed below.

Model

Coach

Scaffold

Articulate

Reflect

Explore

See the *Teaching Hands-on Skills Worksheet* at the end of this section.

REFLECTION QUESTIONS

Be sure to record your answers to these questions in the space provided and file them in the appropriate section of your Professional Development Portfolio.

- What specific hands-on skills will you teach in your course(s)?

_____

_____

_____

_____

_____

- To what other competencies can you apply the Cognitive Apprenticeship teaching strategy?

_____

_____

_____

_____

_____

_____

ESSENTIAL SKILLS FOR WORKPLACE SUCCESS

Summarize the professional skills that students need to have for success in the workplace. Add your own ideas to those listed in the module.

See the *Essential Workplace Skills Idea List* at the end of this section.

REFLECTION QUESTIONS

Be sure to record your answers to these questions in the space provided and file them in the appropriate section of your Professional Development Portfolio.

- What professional skills do your students need in the workplace?

- How can you teach these skills within the context of your course? When and how can students practice these skills?

- What tricks of the trade apply to the content you are teaching?

- What learning or studying strategies do you know? Where could you learn more?

_____

_____

_____

_____

_____

- In what specific ways will students need critical-thinking skills to make good decisions in the workplace? (List as many examples as you can.)

_____

_____

_____

_____

_____

_____

LEARNING ACTIVITIES

The following activities are designed to support you in applying the module concepts to your teaching activities. Use the "Notes for Planning This Activity" spaces to record your ideas and to note resources. Complete each activity and submit as directed by your campus faculty development director. File copies of your activities and any evaluation comments you receive in your Professional Development Portfolio.

Essential Workplace Skills Analysis

Review the course(s) you are teaching and write down a detailed list of the various professional skills that your students need for success in their careers and that you could easily address in your course. Develop additions to your lesson plans and indicate specific ways that you will address these professional skills in each course.

Notes for Planning This Activity:

Student Population Exploration

Make appointments to meet with your supervisor or department head, a student services staff member, and a seasoned instructor who has been teaching in your institution for a few terms. Ask each person to give his or her view of your student population. Concentrate on characteristics that will help you reach your students more effectively. Are there differences in what each person tells you? Why do you think this may be the case?

Notes for Planning This Activity:

Learning and Instructional Theory Research

Go to http://tip.psychology.org and review the many different theories on learning and instruction. Choose one or two theories to explore in more detail and establish a plan to develop your teaching skills by incorporating the elements of the theory into your teaching. Consider selecting a different theory to explore in depth each term so you will constantly be developing your skills.

Notes for Planning This Activity:

Learning Style Discovery

Go to http://www.google.com and conduct a search for "learning style inventory." Select one of the many free online inventories and complete the questions to discover your personal learning style. Complete three or four different inventories to ensure that the results are similar. Next, evaluate the strategies you use or plan to use in your teaching. Are there learning styles potentially represented in your class that you will not address well? Most people teach in the same way that they learn. How can you add teaching strategies to reach the other styles? Write down these ideas in specific places in your teaching notes. Consider assessing each day's class to determine if you have addressed all of the learning styles. Use the results of your assessment to revise your next day's class plan.

Notes for Planning This Activity:

LEARNING OBJECTIVES REVISITED

Review the Learning Objectives for Section 1 and rate your level of achievement for each objective using the rating scale provided. Following your assessment, determine the steps you need to take to meet the objective effectively. For each objective on which you do not rate yourself as a 3, outline a plan of action that you will take to achieve the objective fully. Include a time frame for this plan. Review completed Learning Activities for specific areas in which you need further development. Include the assessment and goals that you write in your Professional Development Portfolio. You may wish to use the Instructor Improvement Plan to set goals to further work toward learning objectives.

1 = did not successfully achieve objective
2 = understand what is needed, but need more study or practice
3 = achieved learning objective thoroughly

	1	2	3
1. The instructor will identify several responsibilities in teaching adults and explain the importance of these responsibilities to the success of the student and the institution.	☐	☐	☐
2. The instructor will be able to describe general characteristics of adult learners and explain specific ways that knowledge of these characteristics can be used to increase the opportunity for learning in classrooms and training facilities.	☐	☐	☐
3. The instructor will be able to describe specific learning and instruction theories and identify specific ways that he or she can use the information to enhance teaching strategies.	☐	☐	☐

STEPS TO ACHIEVE UNMET OBJECTIVES

Steps	Date
1. _____	_____
2. _____	_____
3. _____	_____
4. _____	_____

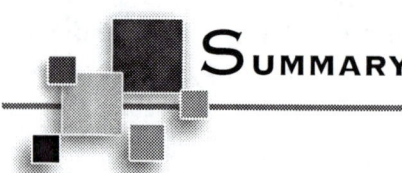

SUMMARY

Section 1 discussed the responsibilities of the instructor or trainer of adult learners emphasizing that there is more to teaching than just presenting information. Instructors have several other responsibilities that impact both student success and institutional success. Additionally, general characteristics that may apply to many adult learners were described with suggestions for effective instructor behaviors that take these characteristics into consideration. Finally, several learning theories were presented briefly with suggestions for using these concepts to help reach individual students. Understanding this information is only the first step in becoming an excellent instructor. It is strongly suggested that instructors commit to enhancing their knowledge about adult learners, developing their instructional skills, and then taking action toward these goals.

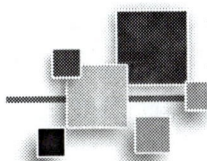

INSTRUCTOR IMPROVEMENT PLAN

Complete the Instructor Improvement Plan for Section 1 at this time. Take the necessary time to prepare a thoughtful, detailed improvement plan. Complete the form and keep it available as you plan and teach your classes for the next few terms. Note your progress, problems, successes, and questions over the next three to six months. At that time, reevaluate the plan and set new goals. Depending on the format you have selected for your Professional Development Portfolio, file the elements of your instructional plan in the appropriate sections. Record the dates for reassessing your goals on the professional development schedule at the beginning of your portfolio.

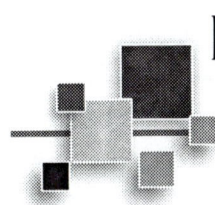

PROFESSIONAL DEVELOPMENT PORTFOLIO ELEMENTS

To finish Section 1, insert your completed responses, reflections, and activities from the section into the designated parts of your Professional Development Portfolio.

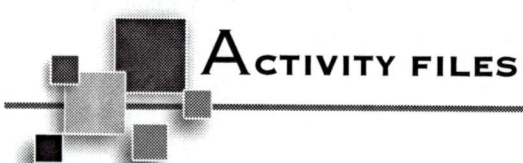

ACTIVITY FILES

The activities on the following pages will help you achieve the Section 1 learning objectives that are referenced throughout the section. In the online module, there are links to PDF files with supporting documents or worksheets for these activities.

ADDRESSING DIFFERENT LEARNING STYLES

 Use the following checklist to ensure that you are addressing all learning styles that may be represented in your class. Add to the list as you think of additional items.

For Visual Learners

- ❏ Use your body language to express emphasis.
- ❏ Use facial expressions to emphasize points, express feelings, and focus student attention.
- ❏ Encourage visual learners to sit close to the front of the class.
- ❏ Use visual displays.
- ❏ Provide students with an outline of your lecture or a list of main topics on the board, in your slides, or in an overhead transparency, and point out each topic as you cover it.
- ❏ Provide a printed lecture outline to help visual learners take notes.
- ❏ Use PowerPoint slides with images, diagrams, and charts.
- ❏ Point out the images and diagrams in the textbook to students.
- ❏ Use flip charts and marker boards.
- ❏ Use videos and movies.
- ❏ Create handouts, especially those with images and diagrams.
- ❏ Use the Internet.
- ❏ Use maps and charts.
- ❏ Allow time in your lectures for visual learners to take detailed notes.
- ❏ Assign activities that require learners to draw, illustrate, or diagram.
- ❏ Describe in detail so that visual learners can form a vivid detailed image.
- ❏ Use activities such as puzzle building, chart making, illustrating or sketching, painting, and fixing things.
- ❏ Ask students to create visual metaphors and to manipulate images.
- ❏ Ask students to design practical objects.
- ❏ Assign presentations where visual learners can present a PowerPoint presentation, poster presentation, or video presentation.
- ❏ Assign projects such as pictorial timelines, project descriptions using pictures, digital camera projects, sketch projects, and so forth.

- ❑ Use learning portfolios to organize student projects.
- ❑ Control the environment for distracting clutter, color, and other visual elements.
- ❑ Dress professionally to avoid distracting visual students.
- ❑ Write down instructions, and use images and diagrams as well as words.
- ❑ Provide a picture or image in a handout as you demonstrate a task.
- ❑ Assign individual projects.
- ❑ Encourage students to use flash cards with both words and pictures or diagrams.
- ❑ Encourage students to use highlighters, symbols, colored pens or pencils, and colored paper.

For Auditory Learners

- ❑ Lecture on complex concepts.
- ❑ Include discussion in your lecture and in small group assignments.
- ❑ Encourage auditory learners to talk about the information they are learning.
- ❑ Assign interviews of industry experts.
- ❑ Use tone, inflection, speed, and other variations in speech to express meaning and emphasize important points.
- ❑ Discuss images as you display them.
- ❑ Talk about the images in the textbook.
- ❑ Allow students to tape record your lectures.
- ❑ Encourage auditory learners to read the text and notes aloud.
- ❑ Assign verbal presentations.
- ❑ Assign peer teaching activities and debates.
- ❑ Control the environment for distracting noise.
- ❑ Give verbal instructions.
- ❑ Talk about what you are doing as you demonstrate a task.

For Kinesthetic Learners

- ❑ Assign hands-on activities.
- ❑ Get students out of their seats for a brief activity during lectures.
- ❑ Hand around equipment, tools, or other tangible items as you discuss concepts.
- ❑ Keep lectures short (less than 20 minutes). Intersperse teaching chunks with hands-on activities.
- ❑ Use experimentation.
- ❑ Simulate the work environment.
- ❑ Assign projects where things are built.
- ❑ Use computer applications.
- ❑ Control the environment for distracting movement.
- ❑ Provide practice time outside of class for hands-on skills.
- ❑ Lecture in a lab environment when possible and use equipment as you talk.
- ❑ Use demonstrations.

BLOOM'S TAXONOMY WORD LIST

 Use the following word list to help you determine the cognitive level at which you teach and assess students. Add to the list as you think of new words that apply.

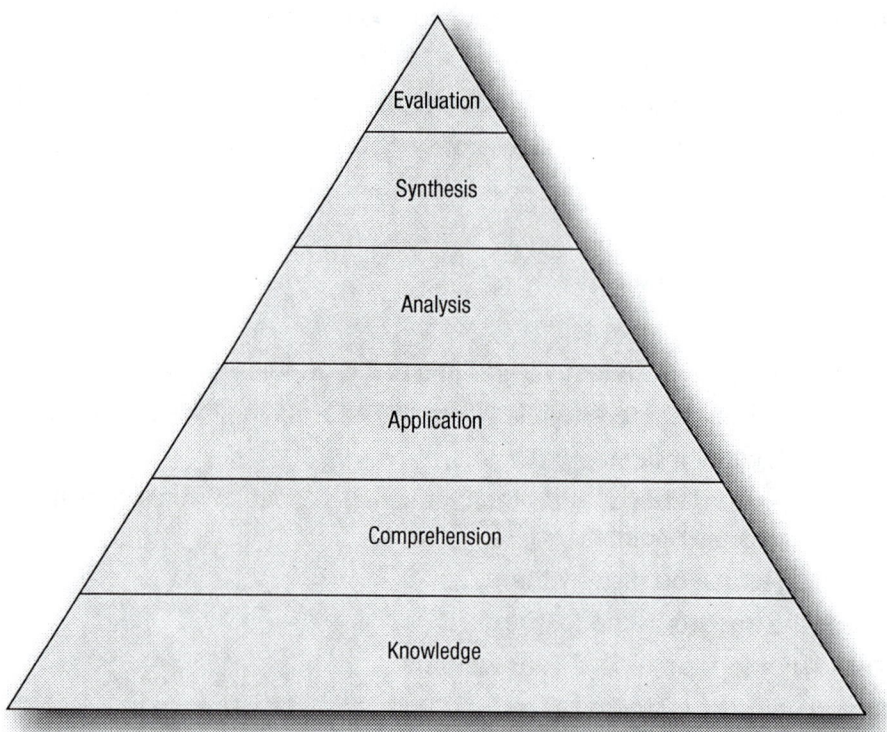

Knowledge—Observe and Recall Facts

list	define	describe	label	collect
examine	identify	tabulate	quote	name
who	when	where	how much	duplicate
arrange	memorize	recognize	relate	recall
repeat	state	reproduce	view	read
cite	count	enumerate	index	study

Comprehension—Understand Information

summarize	describe	interpret	extend	discuss
differentiate	compare	contrast	predict	express
distinguish	estimate	classify	explain	review
indicate	locate	report	restate	make sense of
translate	paraphrase	generalize	site	approximate
understand	trace	give examples	add	detail
associate	characterize	clarify	classify	
elaborate	interpolate			

Application—Use Information

apply	demonstrate	calculate	complete	illustrate
show	solve	examine	modify	relate
change	classify	experiment	discover	choose
dramatize	employ	operate	interpret	practice
schedule	sketch	draw	use	write
assemble	administer	articulate	chart	act
assess	control	determine	implement	instruct
participate	preserve	prepare	teach	project
utilize	transfer	operationalize	produce	acquire
adapt	allocate	assign	attain	avoid
back up	capture	customize	derive	exercise
handle	graph	chart	manipulate	plot
price	round off	sequence	simulate	transcribe

Analysis—Organize Parts

analyze	separate	order	explain	infer
connect	classify	arrange	compare	divide
sort	appraise	criticize	categorize	differentiate
discriminate	distinguish	examine	experiment	question
test	break down	correlate	diagram	focus
illustrate	infer	limit	outline	point out
prioritize	subdivide	transform	audit	characterize
blueprint	confirm	detect	diagnose	dissect
document	file	figure out	group	investigate
lay out	maximize	minimize	proofread	query
train	size up			

Synthesis—Use Old Ideas or Facts to Create New Ideas or Facts

combine	integrate	modify	create	rearrange
substitute	plan	design	develop	invent
compose	formulate	prepare	generalize	what if
rewrite	assemble	collect	compose	construct
manage	organize	set up	prepare	propose
adapt	anticipate	collaborate	devise	express
facilitate	generate	incorporate	initiate	individualize
intervene	integrate	model	negotiate	reconstruct
reorganize	revise	validate	progress	abstract
animate	budget	code	combine	cope

correspond	cultivate	depict	enhance	dictate
generate	handle	import	improve	lecture
network	interface	join	overhaul	portray
prescribe	program	specify	summarize	

Evaluation—Assess Value

rank	grade	assess	evaluate	select
test	measure	recommend	convince	conclude
judge	explain	discriminate	support	defend
compare	summarize	argue	estimate	decide
predict	rate	critique	criticize	fire
interpret	justify	counsel	hire	
validate	verify			

TEACHING HANDS-ON SKILLS

 Use the following questions to help you develop a sound strategy for teaching hands-on skills in your course. Expand these questions as needed to address all issues related to your specific skills.

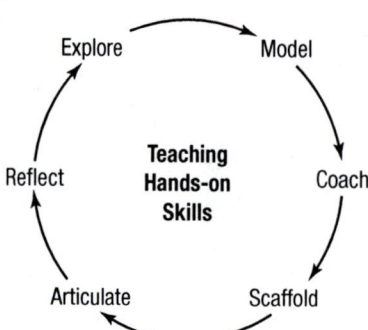

Initial Information

1. What specific skill do you need to teach your students?

_____

_____

2. At what level of proficiency do students need to be able to perform this skill?

_____

_____

3. What specific background information do students need to effectively learn this skill?

_____

_____

_____

4. What equipment is needed?

_____

_____

_____

5. How specifically does the equipment work?

_____

_____

_____

6. Have you completed the activity yourself?

_____

_____

_____

7. What safety precautions are needed for this activity?

_____

_____

_____

8. What professional skills are related to this activity?

_____

_____

_____

Model

1. How specifically should the equipment be set up?

_____

_____

_____

2. What are the safety precautions students should follow in setting up and using the equipment?

_____

_____

_____

3. How will you arrange the room for modeling the skill?

_____

_____

_____

4. Will you provide handouts to help students understand the procedures?

_____

_____

_____

5. Have you allowed time for students to digest the information and ask questions?

_____

_____

_____

6. Does your modeling of the skill simulate the real workplace environment as closely as possible? (If this is not possible, how will you explain the differences to students?)

_____

_____

_____

7. How will you demonstrate the skill? Will you proceed in small chunks, all at once, repeat the steps, etc.?

_____

_____

_____

8. Will you quiz students on their understanding of the proper skill or procedures?

_____

_____

_____

Coach

1. How will you organize your teaching environment so students can practice this skill? Will students work individually or in small groups or take turns completing the skill one at a time in front of the entire class?

_____

_____

_____

2. How will you give feedback to students?

_____

_____

_____

3. Will you encourage students to give each other feedback?

_____

_____

_____

4. What tricks of the trade or hints for optimal performance can you give students?

_____

_____

_____

5. Will you ask probing or critical-thinking questions to students to ensure they understand what they are doing? If so, what are these questions?

_____

_____

_____

6. Will you quiz students on safety issues? What questions will you ask?

_____

_____

_____

7. Will there be an opportunity for you to model the correct behaviors again?

_____

_____

_____

8. Will you provide suggestions on associated professional skills (communication, patient care and interaction, customer service, etc.)?

_____

_____

_____

Scaffold

1. How can you break the skill into small, simple skill-building blocks?

_____

_____

_____

2. In what areas might students be fearful or lack confidence in performing the skill? How could this be a stumbling block for their practice of the skill?

_____

_____

_____

3. How can you reduce or eliminate these fears by making the environment safer or limit the risk or impact of failure?

_____

_____

_____

4. How will you allow for practice of these simple skills?

_____

_____

_____

5. When will you know it is time to combine or expand simple skills?

_____

_____

_____

6. Will you continue to model the big picture skill during this learning process?

_____

_____

_____

7. Will you ask for peer critique during this process?

_____

_____

_____

Articulate

1. How will you ask students to articulate the process of skill acquisition (say it, write it, draw it, teach it, and so forth)?

_____

_____

_____

2. What professional behaviors do you want your students to have as they help each other perform the skill? How do students know about these expectations? Were students involved in creating these expectations?

_____

_____

_____

3. What parts of the skill can students draw or diagram?

_____

_____

_____

4. Is there a diagram or drawing that you can provide to students to assist them?

_____

_____

_____

5. Does the process lend itself to a flow chart, concept map, step-by-step analysis, or other organizational format?

_____

_____

_____

6. What methods can you use to help students understand and remember the skill and its components?

_____

_____

_____

Reflection

1. Have you allowed time for students to reflect on what they are learning?

_____

_____

2. Are there opportunities for additional practice where students can think about the proper techniques?

_____

_____

3. How can students learn to discover flaws in their own performances?

_____

_____

4. Do students have criteria for success to which they can compare their performances and make necessary changes?

_____

_____

5. How can you help students reflect on their learning? What questions can you ask them? How will you deliver these questions?

_____

_____

Exploration

1. What opportunities have you created for students to practice the skill either individually or in groups without your immediate involvement?

_____

_____

_____

2. What safety issues do you need to consider?

_____

_____

_____

3. What issues related to use of supplies should you consider?

_____

_____

_____

4. How will you monitor student performance during this time?

_____

_____

_____

5. When and how will you assess student performance or skill acquisition after they have had an opportunity to acquire the skill and practice it?

_____

_____

_____

6. How will students be able to maintain and improve their skill level throughout and beyond your course?

_____

_____

_____

ESSENTIAL WORKPLACE SKILLS IDEA LIST

Workplace skills are essential to the success of students moving into the workforce as well as to the organization or business in which the student will work as a professional. Employers across the country place a very high priority on the development of these skills. The following idea list represents essential skills for most professionals in most industries. Also included are suggestions for teaching these skills and for providing opportunities for student practice of these skills in and out of the classroom. Consider adding your own thoughts and application ideas to this list as you reflect on your own students and their career success.

Communication Skills

Most students are required to take some form of English fundamentals course, business communication course, speech course, and interpersonal communications course or demonstrate proficiency prior to graduating from college programs. These skills take practice, however, and instructors in all courses have the opportunity to assist students in developing these important skills and to provide an opportunity for practice. In addition, these skills represent excellent learning strategies for students.

Writing

In your classes, consider assigning a variety of writing activities.

- ❏ Ask students to maintain a reflective learning journal throughout the course.
- ❏ Assign students to develop industry-related business documents (memos, letters, proposals, and so forth) as a part of a course-related project.
- ❏ Assign writing an issues paper on an industry-related controversial issue.
- ❏ Assign writing an invented dialogue for a course-related customer, client, or patient dialogue situation. (Ask students to write both an effective dialogue and an ineffective dialogue.)
- ❏ Assign a one-sentence summary of a lecture chunk immediately after the lecture. (This strategy teaches students to be concise and focused.)
- ❏ Ask students to take turns writing class minutes (using a business meeting format).
- ❏ Ask students to do a pre-topic writing assignment. (Students write everything they know about a topic prior to your lecture.)
- ❏ Assign a TV show or video analysis on a topic related to course.
- ❏ Assign students to develop an abstract from a long article. (This strategy teaches students to be concise. Consider using the abstract development guidelines from a professional organization in the field.)

Reading

- ❏ Assign articles or papers to read. Organize students in groups to outline the main points and underlying issues.
- ❏ Create a book club for reading and discussing books related to the course.
- ❏ Assign reading of Internet articles.
- ❏ Ask students to analyze the course textbook and other texts to compare and contrast information and treatment of information. (Your library could maintain comparable textbooks.)

Listening

- ❏ Teach the basics of listening skills and discuss the impact of effective and ineffective listening in the workplace.
- ❏ Develop class listening expectations as a class group.
- ❏ Ask students to develop scenarios where listening skills positively and negatively affect success in the workplace. Discuss in groups.

Presenting

- ❏ Assign presentations on class-related content.
- ❏ Use peer teaching for the teaching of some concepts in class.

Creative Thinking

- ❑ Ask students to invent a new tool or technology to solve an industry problem.
- ❑ Conduct creative small group sessions to solve a problem.
- ❑ Teach students to effectively brainstorm.

Quantitative Reasoning

- ❑ Use a variety of charts, graphs, or quantitative representations of data when possible.
- ❑ Teach students to understand quantitative data using course-related information.
- ❑ Ask students to display data quantitatively.

Problem Solving

- ❑ Provide students with several problems to solve after they have learned the concepts of your course.
- ❑ Ask workplace questions and provide real-life case studies as activities.

Information Gathering

- ❑ Ask questions and assign students to answer them with references from all types of information resources, including the Internet, the library, directories, reference journals, and so forth.
- ❑ Teach students to critique information sources.
- ❑ Critique a Web site related to your field as a group, and then assign additional sites for students to critique in small groups.

Commitment to Learning

- ❑ Ask students to identify several areas related to the topic in your course, but not discussed in class, that they would like to pursue more. Discuss some of these in class.
- ❑ Teach students specific study skills that may facilitate learning of the content in your course. Provide opportunities for students to discuss these skills in small groups.

Career Exploration

- ❑ Provide opportunities for students to shadow professionals in the workplace.
- ❑ Bring in guest speakers to discuss the opportunities in the career.
- ❑ Discuss career opportunities as they relate to specific topics you discuss in class.
- ❑ Discuss licensing, certification, advanced training, and so forth, as they relate to your course.

Other Workplace Skills

There are a variety of other professional skills that every graduate should acquire. The following list represents a few of these skills with ideas for incorporating them into the classroom as projects or learning tools.

Professional Image

- ❑ Sponsor a professional image day where students critique each other in their professional image.
- ❑ Invite image speakers to your class.
- ❑ Discuss the professional image concepts related to your students' careers and the specific impact that excellent and poor image may have on success.
- ❑ Grade students on their professional attitude and interaction in class.
- ❑ Ask students to develop a personal improvement plan to develop their professionalism for success in the workplace.

Time Management

- ❑ Ask students to develop a timeline for their projects and to evaluate these timelines as a group.

Project Management

- ❑ Require students to use established project management strategies in their projects.
- ❑ Discuss the project management strategies and skills related to the concepts you discuss.

Ethics

- ❑ Conduct a brainstorming session on ethical issues related to the topic at hand.
- ❑ Search for industry-related ethics in the news and discuss.

Goal Setting

- ❑ Help students develop goals that relate to their success in the class or their careers.

Computer Applications

- ❑ Require students to use various computer applications (Word, Excel, PowerPoint, statistical packages, and so forth) to complete an assignment.

Safety

- ❑ Conduct a safety analysis of a workplace.
- ❑ Conduct a safety-related interview of a workplace professional.
- ❑ Assign students to research safety regulations related to the topics of your course.

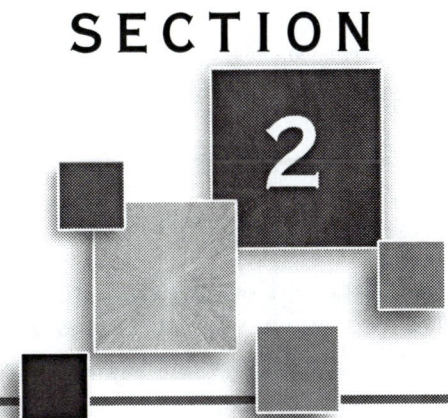
PREPARING TO TEACH AND THE FIRST DAYS OF CLASS

LEARNING OBJECTIVES

Upon successful completion of Section 2, the instructor will have achieved the following objectives. Check off each of the objectives as you have mastered it. You will have the opportunity to assess your performance on each objective at the end of Section 2.

4. The instructor will be able to identify the various paperwork responsibilities that may be required and why each is important.
5. The instructor will be able to go through a detailed process to select and review a textbook for a course according to established procedures at the school.
6. The instructor will be able to develop an informative course syllabus for a course.
7. The instructor will be able to identify important characteristics of effective and professional handouts to help students learn the content presented in a course.
8. The instructor will be able to develop a major learning activity using an Activity Development Worksheet.
9. The instructor will be able to organize a grade book.
10. The instructor will be able to review a course to determine the facility, equipment, and instructional technology needs and address scheduling considerations.
11. The instructor will be able to establish the goals and agenda for the first day of class.
12. The instructor will be able to design an ice-breaking activity for the first day of class.

INTRODUCTORY QUESTIONS

- What are the different areas in which you must prepare for a successful class start?
- How specifically can lack of preparation cost time later in the course?
- How specifically can proper preparation save time later in the course?
- What are your goals during the first days of class?
- How might meeting these goals or not meeting these goals affect the entire course?
- What elements should be included in a course syllabus?

- What are common flaws in handouts used in class?
- What are an instructor's options for resources other than traditional textbooks?

OVERVIEW

Section 2 provides ideas for preparing for teaching a course and conducting the first days of class. Organization, preparation, review of course content, and first day activities are all discussed with ideas for making these activities easy and organized. The section suggests several specific ideas that can be immediately implemented.

SUGGESTED GENERAL GUIDELINES: PREPARATION AND THE FIRST DAY OF CLASS

Summarize the importance of organization and planning for the first day of class.

REFLECTION QUESTIONS

Be sure to record your answers to these questions in the space provided and file them in the appropriate section of your Professional Development Portfolio.

- How would you rate your organizational skills on a scale of 1 to 10 where 1 is highly disorganized and 10 is highly organized?

_____

_____

_____

_____

_____

- In what areas are you strong? Weak?

_____

_____

_____

_____

_____

ADMINISTRATIVE PAPERWORK

Note the importance of completing required administrative paperwork in a timely manner. For each of the headings below, note important documents and note any additional information that will be useful to you.

Complete and Submit Employment Paperwork

Complete and Submit Accrediting Body Paperwork

Review Other Information Related to Your Course

REFLECTION QUESTIONS

Be sure to record your answers to these questions in the space provided and file them in the appropriate section of your Professional Development Portfolio.

- What paperwork is required by your institution or department? Have you completed all of this information and submitted it appropriately?

_____

_____

_____

_____

_____

TEXTBOOK SELECTION AND REVIEW

Summarize the textbook selection process at your institution. Record any questions or concerns that you can pose to the appropriate administrator.

GENERAL STRATEGIES FOR TEXTBOOK SELECTION AND REVIEW

Use the Textbook Selection Checklist as a guide to assessing a textbook. See the *Textbook Selection Checklist* at the end of this section.

Using the questions in the online module, review the textbook selected for your course and note important aspects of the text.

REFLECTION QUESTIONS

Be sure to record your answers to these questions in the space provided and file them in the appropriate section of your Professional Development Portfolio.

- What features in a textbook do you expect or like to see? Why?

_____

_____

_____

_____

_____

- How do you think students should best utilize their textbook for study?

_____

_____

_____

_____

_____

- What features in a textbook do you like to avoid, if you have a choice?

_____

_____

_____

_____

_____

- How can you turn textbook weaknesses or errors into opportunities for student learning?

_____

_____

_____

_____

_____

DEVELOPMENT OF COURSE MATERIALS

List the tasks you are expected to complete to develop course material. If material is provided for you, note where you can retrieve it.

Developing the Syllabus

Briefly discuss the importance of the syllabus. Note institutional policies to consider when creating a syllabus.

GENERAL STRATEGIES FOR DEVELOPING THE SYLLABUS

From the bulleted items in the module, list the elements that you need to include in your syllabus.

See the *Course Syllabus Template Example* at the end of this section.

Developing Course Handouts

Briefly summarize the importance of creating useful handouts.

GENERAL STRATEGIES FOR DEVELOPING EFFECTIVE HANDOUTS

Summarize each of the bulleted points for creating a well-designed and useful handout.

REFLECTION QUESTIONS

Be sure to record your answers to these questions in the space provided and file them in the appropriate section of your Professional Development Portfolio.

- What characteristics of handouts frustrate you? (Think back to courses you have taken.)

_____

_____

_____

_____

_____

- What do you like to see in handouts in a course you take?

_____

_____

_____

_____

_____

Developing Learning Activities

Summarize the importance of developing class activities at the beginning of the course.

GENERAL STRATEGIES FOR DEVELOPING LEARNING ACTIVITIES

Summarize each of the elements that contribute to an effective learning activity.

See the *Activity Development Worksheet* at the end of this section.

REFLECTION QUESTIONS

Be sure to record your answers to these questions in the space provided and file them in the appropriate section of your Professional Development Portfolio.

- What are the best activities you have ever conducted or participated in? Why were they so good?

_____

_____

_____

_____

_____

- What are the worst activities you have ever conducted or participated in? Why were they so bad?

_____

_____

_____

_____

_____

GRADE BOOK ORGANIZATION

Explain the benefits of creating and organizing your grade book before the course begins.

GENERAL STRATEGIES FOR DEVELOPING AND MAINTAINING A GRADE BOOK

Summarize each bulleted point regarding creating a grade book. Note strategies that you believe to be especially helpful. Add additional strategies that you think of.

Electronic Grade Books

Review the suggested Web sites and note the features of electronic grade books that you find helpful.

REFLECTION QUESTIONS

Be sure to record your answers to these questions in the space provided and file them in the appropriate section of your Professional Development Portfolio.

- Think back to courses you have taught or participated in as a student. What were frustrations you had in grading?

- What strategies made the grading process difficult or frustrating?

- What strategies made the grading process work well?

EQUIPMENT, FACILITY, AND INSTRUCTIONAL TECHNOLOGIES

What equipment will you need for your course? What are the procedures for obtaining equipment at your institution?

GENERAL STRATEGIES FOR OBTAINING AND USING INSTRUCTIONAL EQUIPMENT

Note the steps and important considerations for obtaining and using instructional equipment.

See the *Equipment, Facility, and Instructional Technology Worksheet* at the end of this section.

THE FIRST DAY OF CLASS

Summarize the significance of the first day of class.

GENERAL STRATEGIES FOR HAVING A SUCCESSFUL FIRST DAY

Note each strategy for maximizing the success of the first day of class. Note how each strategy can be customized to meet your needs and those of your students.

Preparing for the First Day

Briefly discuss the importance of being organized for the first day. Consider the benefits to students as well as to you as an instructor.

GENERAL STRATEGIES FOR ORGANIZING FOR THE FIRST DAY

For each of the strategies listed in the module, note ideas for incorporating each into your first day of class.

See the *Sample First Day Agenda Form* at the end of this section.

TAKE IT TO THE CLASSROOM ACTIVITIES

Take It to the Classroom activities are designed to support you in applying the module's concepts to the classroom. Course objectives will be met most effectively and learning will be most beneficial if the activities are completed in conjunction with the material found in the online course.

In addition to reviewing your syllabus and beginning to cover the course content (both of which will depend on your individual situation), you can use additional activities to increase interaction within the class and to establish rapport between class members. Consider the following introductory activities to develop a feeling of community in your class.

Student Information Sheets

Ask students to fill out student information sheets with basic identifying information and information that will help you understand your students better. Include important things that are currently going on in their lives, if and where they are working and how many hours each week they work, a description of their family or home life, and other responsibilities that will occupy their time during the course. Remember to respect confidentiality.

Notes for Planning This Activity:

Students' Initial Feelings

Ask students to write their initial feelings about the course on a piece of paper. Then, ask volunteers to read what they wrote and encourage a discussion. Generally, students have many of the same feelings. Consider listing the responses on the board and as a group, discussing ways to capitalize on positive feelings and alleviate any negative ones. Alternatively, ask students to hand the papers in anonymously and then tally the comments on the board. In this way, commonalities are obvious, but the approach may feel safer for students.

Notes for Planning This Activity:

Instructor's Initial Feelings

Ask students to write down what you as the instructor might be feeling on the first day of class. Ask for volunteers to share their comments, and then discuss your own feelings. This often helps students to realize that you are a typical person just like themselves. Consider listing the responses on the board and as a group, discussing the feelings. Consider completing this activity in conjunction with the Students' Initial Feelings activity and review similarities and differences between instructor and students.

Notes for Planning This Activity:

Student Questions

Start the traditional introduction process, but allow students to ask up to five questions of each classmate. This technique can be very entertaining and informative. Of course, students retain the right to choose not to answer a question.

Notes for Planning This Activity:

People Scavenger Hunt

Conduct a "People Scavenger Hunt." Create a list of descriptors of people and make copies for each student. Examples of descriptors are "someone who has taught a course," "someone who works and goes to school," and "someone who has at least two children under 3 years old." Formulate statements that reveal students' expertise, current family or work situations, educational backgrounds, or interests. Allow students a specified amount of time to find classmates who match the descriptors and fill in the statements with student names. Share the results in the large group.

Notes for Planning This Activity:

Information Exchange

Encourage students to exchange phone numbers, e-mail addresses, etc., and to seek out study groups or partners or other students who will take notes for them if they miss class.

Notes for Planning This Activity:

"No One Has Done This"

Ask students to introduce themselves and state something they have done that they believe no one else in the class has done. This usually makes for interesting or entertaining conversation.

Notes for Planning This Activity:

Predictions

Supply the students with a list of questions to be used to get to know each other. Examples include, "What are your hobbies?", "What pets do you have and what are their names?", and "What is your best subject and why?" Organize students into pairs.

Instruct students to take turns asking their partners about the topics. The partner is silent and the student asking the questions must predict the answers. The positions are then reversed. When completed, students introduce their partners to the class using the predictions they have made. The student being introduced then corrects the predictions with the truth.

Notes for Planning This Activity:

True or False

Instruct each person to write down five things about themselves on a piece of paper. Three of these should be true and two should be false. The class as a whole decides which is false and which is true.

Notes for Planning This Activity:

Three Things in Common

Instruct students to form pairs and to find three things they have in common. Introduce each other to the class and state the three things in common.

Notes for Planning This Activity:

Find the Person

Instruct each person to write three things about themselves on an index card. Gather the cards and distribute them randomly to the class ensuring that no one gets his or her own card. Have students try to find the person that matches the card. Have students introduce the person who matches the card to the entire group.

Notes for Planning This Activity:

REFLECTION QUESTIONS

Be sure to record your answers to these questions in the space provided and file them in the appropriate section of your Professional Development Portfolio.

- What were your biggest fears or concerns as a student on the first day of class?

_____

_____

_____

_____

_____

- What did your instructors do or not do to alleviate these fears?

_____

_____

_____

_____

_____

- What did your instructors do or not do to create more concern about the course?

_____

_____

_____

_____

_____

- What introduction activities have you used in workshops, courses, or seminars that you enjoyed?

_____

_____

_____

_____

_____

LEARNING ACTIVITIES

The following activities are designed to support you in applying the module concepts to your teaching activities. Use the "Notes for Planning This Activity" spaces to record your ideas and to note resources. Complete each activity and submit as directed by your campus faculty development director. File copies of your activities and any evaluation comments you receive in your Professional Development Portfolio.

Syllabus Comparison

Evaluate a syllabus that you currently use against the criteria listed in Section 2. Evaluate your current syllabus for elements that you find to be effective and note those that can be improved. Incorporate changes into the syllabus the next time you teach the course. If your school provides you with a standard template, be sure to go through the proper channels to revise the document.

Notes for Planning This Activity:

Handout Review

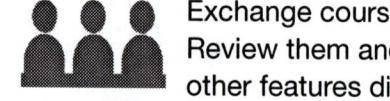

Exchange course handouts with other instructors in your department. Review them and exchange feedback on their clarity, professionalism, and other features discussed in Section 2. Brainstorm ways the handouts can be improved, based on the criteria provided in Section 2.

Notes for Planning This Activity:

Ice Breakers

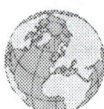

Conduct an Internet search for ice-breaker activities. Many sites contain ideas for these kinds of activities. Develop a list of additional ideas that you might like to try for your course.

Notes for Planning This Activity:

LEARNING OBJECTIVES REVISITED

Review the Learning Objectives for Section 2 and rate your level of achievement for each objective using the rating scale provided. Following your assessment, determine the steps you need to take to meet the objective effectively. For each objective on which you do not rate yourself as a 3, outline a plan of action that you will take to achieve the objective fully. Include a time frame for this plan. Review completed Learning Activities for specific areas in which you need further development. Include the assessment and goals that you write in your Professional Development Portfolio. You may wish to use the Instructor Improvement Plan to set goals to further work toward learning objectives.

1 = did not successfully achieve objective
2 = understand what is needed, but need more study or practice
3 = achieved learning objective thoroughly

	1	2	3
4. The instructor will be able to identify the various paperwork responsibilities that may be required and why each is important.	☐	☐	☐
5. The instructor will be able to go through a detailed process to select and review a textbook for a course according to established procedures at the school.	☐	☐	☐
6. The instructor will be able to develop an informative course syllabus for a course.	☐	☐	☐
7. The instructor will be able to identify important characteristics of effective and professional handouts to help students learn the content presented in a course.	☐	☐	☐
8. The instructor will be able to develop a major learning activity using an Activity Development Worksheet.	☐	☐	☐
9. The instructor will be able to organize a grade book.	☐	☐	☐
10. The instructor will be able to review a course to determine the facility, equipment, and instructional technology needs and address scheduling considerations.	☐	☐	☐
11. The instructor will be able to establish the goals and agenda for the first day of class.	☐	☐	☐
12. The instructor will be able to design an ice-breaking activity for the first day of class.	☐	☐	☐

STEPS TO ACHIEVE UNMET OBJECTIVES

Steps	Date
1. _____	_____
2. _____	_____
3. _____	_____
4. _____	_____

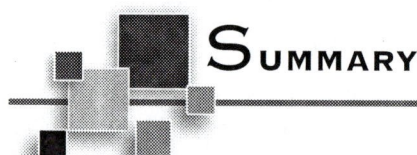

SUMMARY

Section 2 discussed the importance of preparation and organization of the many tasks required by the instructor prior to the start of a class. Recommendations include completing the administrative paperwork required for teaching a course, selecting and reviewing the textbook for the course, developing the course syllabus, developing professional handouts and appropriate learning activities for the course, setting up the grade book, and designing your agenda for that important first day of class. Taking the appropriate amount of time to effectively prepare for the course saves huge amounts of time throughout the course and helps to establish the expectations and tone you desire for students.

INSTRUCTOR IMPROVEMENT PLAN

Complete the Instructor Improvement Plan for Section 2 at this time. Take the necessary time to prepare a thoughtful, detailed improvement plan. Complete the form and keep it available as you plan and teach your classes for the next few terms. Note your progress, problems, successes, and questions over the next three to six months. At that time, reevaluate the plan and set new goals. Depending on the format you have selected for your Professional Development Portfolio, file the elements of your instructional plan in the appropriate sections. Record the dates for reassessing your goals on the professional development schedule at the beginning of your portfolio.

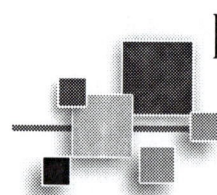

PROFESSIONAL DEVELOPMENT PORTFOLIO ELEMENTS

To finish Section 2, insert your completed responses, reflections, and activities from the section into the designated parts of your Professional Development Portfolio.

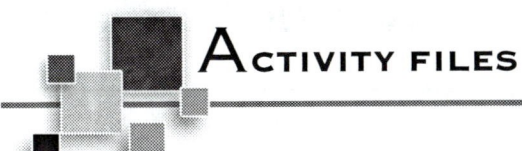

ACTIVITY FILES

The activities on the following pages will help you achieve the Section 2 learning objectives that are referenced throughout the section. In the online module, there are links to PDF files with supporting documents or worksheets for these activities.

TEXTBOOK SELECTION CHECKLIST

Talk with your department colleagues and identify your textbook publisher representative. Make contact and discuss the various resources and supplements that are associated with your text. If you are required to choose your textbook, contact the representatives from several publishers and ask that they send or bring you appropriate selections for you to review. Use this checklist to help identify the best choice.

TEXTBOOK CRITERIA	YES	NO	COMMENTS
1. Does the textbook address a majority of the topics you must cover in your class?			
2. Does the textbook cover the topics in the appropriate depth?			
3. Is the reading level appropriate for your students?			
4. Often, chapters begin with outcomes or chapter objectives. Do these correlate with the objectives of your course?			
5. Do the headings/subheadings and other design features make the text easy to read, study, and review?			
6. Is the content cohesive throughout the text? How can you tell this?			
7. Is the design logical and consistent?			
8. Does the author provide suggestions for using the textbook?			
9. Does the content cover current material, including laws, technology, procedures, industry issues, and so forth?			
10. Does the content cover diversity issues related to the industry and topics?			
11. Is the text written so it is culturally sensitive, meaning that it avoids slang, ethnic stereotyping, political incorrectness, one-culture references, and so forth?			

TEXTBOOK CRITERIA	YES	NO	COMMENTS
12. Does the content relate to the workplace?			
13. Does the book utilize several kinds of learning tools, including end-of-chapter questions, self-tests, case studies, activities, and so forth?			
14. Are answers to the chapter questions or problems provided to allow students to test their understanding of the material?			
15. Do the chapters begin with a summary or outline?			
16. Do the chapters end with a follow-up summary?			
17. Do the images, diagrams, charts, and other visual elements help students to understand the content?			
18. Are the figures and tables clearly labeled, organized, and well presented?			
19. Does the text avoid clutter, busy work, unnecessary elements or images, or other distractions?			
20. Does the textbook include sidebars, reflective questions, trivia, factual boxes, bulleted lists, or some other element to add interest to the text and engage the readers?			
21. Is there a glossary of terms at the end of the textbook?			
22. Is there an index to help readers find information within the text?			
23. Are the references used current and representative of accepted resources for your industry?			
24. Are there supplemental resources that correlate to the textbook such as workbooks, case study collections, solutions manuals, instructor manuals, detailed lesson plans or curricula, image libraries, CD-ROMs or Web sites containing electronic resources, and so forth?			
25. Is the cost of the textbook and other required resources reasonable for your students?			

COURSE SYLLABUS TEMPLATE EXAMPLE

Use this syllabus template or acquire the standard course syllabus for your institution and course. Develop the syllabus for your course or review the existing course syllabus and make any necessary changes. Ensure that all dates, grades, and other changeable information have been revised.

Course Syllabus

Course Title:
Course Number:
Course Section:
Time and Date:
Term:

Prerequisites to Course:

Course Resources:
   Textbook: (Required)

   Workbook: (Optional)

   Lab Manual: (Required)

Equipment and Supplies:

Instructor:
   Phone: **E-mail:**   **Fax:**
   Office Location:
   Office Hours:

Lab Assistant:
   Phone: **E-mail:**   **Fax:**
   Office Location:
   Office Hours:

Teaching Assistant:
   Phone: **E-mail:**   **Fax:**
   Office Location:
   Office Hours:

Course Overview:

Learning Objectives/Competencies:

   1.
   2.

3.

4.

5.

Course Policies and Procedures:

Attendance, Absences, and Tardiness:

Make-up Work:

Late Submission:

Incomplete Grades:

Withdrawal:

Safety Considerations:

Ethics, Academic Dishonesty, Professionalism, and Behavior Expectations:

Financial Considerations:

Participation:

Lab Procedures and Expectations:

Lab Practice Opportunities and Lab Hours:

Evaluation:

Students with Special Needs:

Course Schedule and Calendar:

WEEK	ASSIGNMENT	DUE DATE

ACTIVITY DEVELOPMENT WORKSHEET

 This worksheet is intended to provide a guide for creating meaningful and relevant activities for your adult students. Make as many copies of this worksheet as needed to thoughtfully develop activities for your class.

❏ **Purpose of Activity**
— Why are you doing this activity in the first place?
— Is there a better way for students to learn material?
— How does it relate to the course?
— How does it relate to the program of study?
— How does it relate to career success?

❏ **Learning Objectives**
— What specific learning objective(s) does the activity address?
— What content knowledge should students achieve?
— What technical skills should students achieve?
— What professional skills should students achieve?
— How do students know this?

❏ **Background Information Required**
— What prior information is needed?
— What assignments must be completed?
— What knowledge and skills from previous courses must be recalled?
— How will you assess if students have learned this?
— Do students understand required professional skills?

❏ **Useful Resources**
— What should students read prior to the activity?
— Is there a specific textbook section?
— Are there articles, Web sites, videos, audiotapes, and so forth available for review?
— How will you assess if students have completed preparation?

❏ **Detailed Instructions**
— What exactly are students supposed to do in order to complete the activity?
— Are the instructions clear?
— Has equipment been considered?
— Do instructions work?
— Is the amount of detail appropriate for the objectives of the activity?

❏ **Equipment**
— Have you reserved the equipment/facilities needed for the activity?
— Do you know how to operate the equipment?
— Have you checked the equipment recently to ensure that it is in working order?
— Have you planned for the worst case scenario related to equipment?
— Do you have the appropriate type and amount of supplies needed?
— Will students work in groups or individually?
— Have you organized the appropriate amount of equipment and supplies for the number of groups or individuals in your class?
— How will you organize the groups?

❏ **Criteria for Success**
— What criteria determine successful completion of the activity?
— How will students know this?
— Does assessment correlate closely with criteria for success?
— Do criteria correlate closely with industry standards (certification, workplace expectations, etc.)?

❏ **Evaluation**
— How will you evaluate students?
— How will students know?
— Will all elements of activity be evaluated (content, skills, professional skills)?
— Will students evaluate each other?
— If students work in groups, is evaluation equitable?

❏ **Opportunities for Practice**
— If skills are involved, will students have additional opportunities for practice?
— Do students know exactly what they need to work on?
— Have you provided sufficient feedback to allow for effective practice?

❏ **Student Self-Assessment**
— How can students assess their own progress (content, skill, and professional skill)?
— Have you included self-assessment in the activity itself?
— Are there opportunities for peer assessment?
— Will self- or peer assessment be included in any grade?

❏ **Critical-Thinking Activities**
— What specific critical-thinking skills should students develop or practice?
— What specific critical-thinking activities are included?
— What critical-thinking questions will you ask? When?
— How will you facilitate critical thinking in groups?

❏ **Critique of Activity**
— Have you allowed students to critique the activity itself?
— How will you critique this activity for improvement areas?
— How will you include comments into activities?

EQUIPMENT, FACILITY, AND INSTRUCTIONAL TECHNOLOGY WORKSHEET

Use this worksheet to plan the equipment and other supplies that you will need to successfully complete your planned classroom activities. Include pertinent information, such as deadlines for reserving equipment, special orders or requests, or other details to which you will need to attend. Refer to this frequently to ensure that you are effectively prepared for your classes. Note that "Plan B" ideas give you the opportunity to have a backup agenda—just in case.

DATE/DAY	OBJECTIVE	ACTIVITY DESCRIPTION	FACILITY NEEDED	EQUIPMENT NEEDED	SUPPLIES NEEDED	PLAN B IDEAS

SAMPLE FIRST DAY AGENDA

Use this sample agenda as a guide for developing the agenda for the first day of each of the courses you teach. Specifically write down how you will set the tone and expectations for your course and how you will motivate your students to be excited about the coming term.

TOPIC	DETAIL	ACTIVITY
Welcome to the Course	Welcome students to the course and introduce yourself.	
Course Syllabus and Policies	Go over each element of the syllabus. Discuss the expectations of the students in terms of behavior. Go over policies.	Hand out the course syllabus. Facilitate discussion to allow students to have input on expectations and policies.
Course Calendar	Go over the schedule of the course including major activities.	Hand out any information you have on the activities of the course. Hand out a calendar of the course, if it is not in the syllabus.
Textbook and Other Course Materials	Go over the textbook thoroughly and discuss ways students can use it effectively for your course. Cover the additional supplements.	Have a copy of your textbook and all supplements in case some students have not purchased it.
Introductions and Ice Breaker	Use an ice-breaking activity to help students feel comfortable and get to know each other.	Conduct an ice-breaking activity.
Lab or Shop Tour	Explain the lab, shop, or library including the major equipment, policies, and hours.	Take a tour of the lab, shop, or library.
Study Tips	Discuss ideas for studying effectively for your course.	Facilitate a study strategy discussion.
Lecture on Topic #1	Lecture on your first topic.	Conduct an appropriate activity to engage learners.

SECTION 3

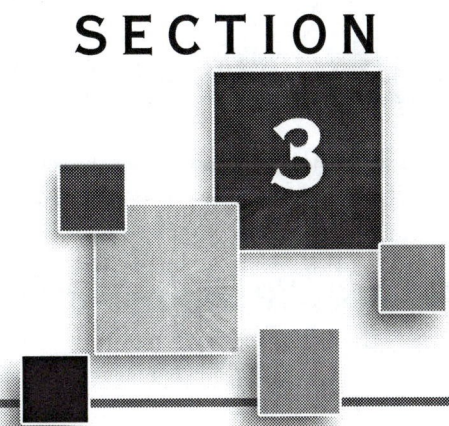

THE DAY-TO-DAY CLASSROOM ENVIRONMENT

LEARNING OBJECTIVES

Upon successful completion of Section 3, the instructor will have achieved the following objectives. Check off each of the objectives as you have mastered it. You will have the opportunity to assess your performance on each objective at the end of Section 3.

13. The instructor will be able to develop an effective and interesting lecture appropriate for a specific learner population.
14. The instructor will identify effective listening skills and evaluate his or her own skills related to listening to students.
15. The instructor will identify effective questioning techniques and positive ways to field student questions.
16. The instructor will identify skills needed to facilitate effective discussions in the classroom, both in large and small group situations.
17. The instructor will be able to explain the importance of active learning in the classroom and demonstrate the ability to develop these types of activities for class.

INTRODUCTORY QUESTIONS

- What are the specific tasks and responsibilities you have as an instructor in the day-to-day classroom?
- What are the specific skills instructors need to complete these tasks successfully and to meet their daily classroom responsibilities?

OVERVIEW

Section 3 provides an overview of day-to-day classroom activities, including presentations and lectures, discussion and questioning, activities, and homework. Topics include tips on classroom presentation, lecture, discussion, asking questions, and methods for incorporating active learning into the teaching strategies.

SUGGESTED GENERAL GUIDELINES: IMPORTANCE OF DAY-TO-DAY CLASSROOM OPERATIONS

Based on the information in the online module, summarize each of the following strategies for maximizing the success of day-to-day operations in the classroom.

Establish Strong Professional Relationships With Students

Choose Your Teaching Format Thoughtfully

Plan Carefully and Thoroughly

Use Best Practices

ESTABLISH RAPPORT

Define rapport and describe what it means to establish rapport with students.

GENERAL STRATEGIES FOR ESTABLISHING RAPPORT

Summarize each strategy for establishing rapport in your classroom. Add your own ideas to the list from the online module.

See the *Instructor Characteristics Rating Sheet* at the end of this section.

REFLECTION QUESTIONS

Be sure to record your answers to these questions in the space provided and file them in the appropriate section of your Professional Development Portfolio.

- What characteristics do you respect in people whom you have had as leaders or instructors?

_____

_____

_____

_____

_____

- What causes you to lose respect for people?

_____

_____

_____

_____

_____

- If you were a student in your class, how would you rate yourself as an instructor? Why?

_____

_____

_____

_____

_____

- What might you do to increase your respect rating?

_____

_____

_____

_____

_____

BE AN EXCELLENT LECTURER

Briefly describe the importance of developing effective lecture skills.

```
┌─────────────────────────────────────────┐
│                                         │
│                                         │
│                                         │
└─────────────────────────────────────────┘
```

GENERAL STRATEGIES FOR DELIVERING EFFECTIVE LECTURES

Summarize each strategy for delivering an effective lecture. Add additional suggestions based on your experience.

■ ■ ■ DIVERSITY CONSIDERATIONS ■ ■ ■

When giving a lecture, be aware that some students may have trouble with verbal delivery of information for a number of reasons. Some examples include students who may be hearing impaired or students for whom English is a second language. Be aware of students who might have difficulty understanding and work with them to make effective and reasonable accommodations.

DIVERSITY REFLECTIONS

- What are some strategies for providing information in an alternative format for students who may have difficulty utilizing verbal delivery of information?

_____

_____

_____

_____

_____

GENERAL STRATEGIES FOR USING LECTURE EFFECTIVELY

Based on the information in the module, summarize each of the following strategies for using lecture effectively. Tailor your responses to include what you can do to develop your skills in the listed area.

Be Professional in Appearance and Behavior

Make Sure Your Material Is Well-Organized

Limit Lectures to 15 to 20 Minutes

Limit Lectures to Three or Four Points

Facilitate Learning Rather Than Present the Material

Avoid Lecturing Strictly from Notes

Move Around in Your Class

Pay Attention to All Students

Continuously Monitor Students' Progress in Class

REFLECTION QUESTIONS

Be sure to record your answers to these questions in the space provided and file them in the appropriate section of your Professional Development Portfolio.

- Assess the lecture notes you have developed for your course (or think about developing these lecture notes). What elements discussed on the preceding pages might you need to add to your lesson plans?

_____

_____

_____

_____

_____

- What elements discussed on the preceding pages do you do really well?

_____

_____

_____

_____

_____

- Are there other elements not discussed that you think would improve your lectures?

_____

_____

_____

_____

_____

Take It to the Classroom activities are designed to support you in applying the module's concepts to the classroom. Course objectives will be met most effectively and learning will be most beneficial if the activities are completed in conjunction with the material found in the online course.

Instructors can use many techniques to develop lecturing skills and improve their lectures. Consider the following suggestions for activities to successfully use lecture in your classroom.

PowerPoint Presentations

Create a PowerPoint presentation for a lecture that you have planned. (Make sure that you have access to an LCD projector or other form of projection. If not, consider making overhead transparencies from printouts of the PowerPoint slides.) Use the presentation to supplement your lecture. Note how the PowerPoint presentation enhances your teaching, and note any slides you wish to change.

Notes for Planning This Activity:

Mini-Quizzes

To assess students' understanding of lecture content, give "quizzes" over lecture material. Instead of grading the quizzes, use the responses as a basis for discussion of the material and an assessment of where students might need review. Inform students of the purpose of the "quiz" and encourage them to use it as a tool for developing their learning.

Notes for Planning This Activity:

Lecture Organization Tool

Create a lecture organization tool that fits your teaching needs and style. One method is to create a form that can be printed and completed by hand for each lecture. Other instructors prefer an electronic document that allows insertion of other files and information. It is important to select a method that suits your preferences and that you will use consistently. Develop and refine the tool as you use it.

Notes for Planning This Activity:

Variations on Lectures

List the suggestions for variations on lecture. Note those that would be effective alternatives in your classes. Jot down ideas for each activity you would like to try.

REFLECTION QUESTIONS

Be sure to record your answers to these questions in the space provided and file them in the appropriate section of your Professional Development Portfolio.

- For the courses you are or will be teaching, what techniques will you use to capture your students' attention for each topic?

- How can you keep your students' attention?

- Do you think that some students will be engaged by different strategies? How so?

_____

_____

_____

_____

_____

BE AN EXCELLENT COMMUNICATOR

Describe the benefits of being an excellent communicator in the classroom.

Listening

Summarize the multiple facets of listening that enable an instructor to communicate effectively with students.

GENERAL STRATEGIES FOR DEVELOPING LISTENING SKILLS

Summarize each of the following strategies for developing listening skills. For each, note what you can do to develop your listening skills.

Develop the Habit of Listening and the Willingness to Listen to Students

Allow Students to Complete Their Thoughts

Give Time to Students to Process What They Are Saying and Verbalize Their Thoughts

Keep the Focus on the Student

Be Respectful of the Opinions and Perspectives of Others

Demonstrate That You Are Listening with Supportive Mannerisms and Body Language

REFLECTION QUESTIONS

Be sure to record your answers to these questions in the space provided and file them in the appropriate section of your Professional Development Portfolio.

- What makes you feel that you are being listened to? (Describe specific ways in as much detail as you can.)

_____

_____

_____

_____

_____

- What makes you feel that you are not being listened to? (Describe specific ways in as much detail as you can.)

_____

_____

_____

_____

_____

- What are the results of each of the above situations? How do you think students respond to each of the above situations? (Be as specific as possible.)

_____

_____

_____

_____

_____

_____

EFFECTIVE QUESTIONING

Summarize the benefits of effective questioning in the classroom, as discussed in the online module.

> ## GENERAL STRATEGIES FOR EFFECTIVE QUESTIONING
>
> Summarize each of the following suggestions for effective questioning. For each, note actions you can take to develop your questioning skills.

Plan Your Questions Prior to Class

Create Questions in Line with Your Course Objectives

See the *Bloom's Taxonomy Word List* at the end of Section 1.

Ask More Open-Ended Questions in Your Class Than Closed-Ended Questions

Train Students to Answer Questions

Never Make Students Uncomfortable With Questions

Give Students Time to Answer

Solicit Questions from Students

Acknowledge Students for Asking and Answering Questions

■ ■ ■ DIVERSITY CONSIDERATIONS ■ ■ ■

Be aware that in some cultures, instructors are viewed as authority figures, and it is considered rude to question or disagree with an authority figure. A student from a culture of this nature may appear uninvolved in discussion sessions. Make an effort to understand the student's perspective. With the student's input, devise a way to involve him or her in a way that is compatible with his or her cultural orientation.

DIVERSITY REFLECTIONS

- How would you involve a student who is reluctant to ask questions in the class activities and discussions?

REFLECTION QUESTIONS

Be sure to record your answers to these questions in the space provided and file them in the appropriate section of your Professional Development Portfolio.

- How often do you ask questions in class? (Analyze your teaching to determine how many questions you ask.)

- At what cognitive level are your questions? Are they closed-ended or open-ended? Are they higher on the Bloom's taxonomy pyramid or lower?

_____

_____

_____

_____

_____

- How do your questions reflect the learning objectives of your course?

_____

_____

_____

_____

_____

FACILITATING DISCUSSION

Summarize the benefits of classroom discussion for students.

GENERAL STRATEGIES FOR FACILITATING DISCUSSION

Summarize each of the following strategies for facilitating discussion in the class-room. Note what you can do to develop your own facilitation skills.

Teach Students How to Discuss

Let Students Participate in Establishing Discussion Guidelines

Plan Discussions Thoughtfully

Teach Students How to Think Critically and Creatively Prior to Starting the Discussion

Manage the Students Effectively

REFLECTION QUESTIONS

Be sure to record your answers to these questions in the space provided and file them in the appropriate section of your Professional Development Portfolio.

- Think back to previous courses you have taught or taken as a student. What was the optimal discussion situation?

_____

_____

_____

_____

_____

- What were the characteristics and behaviors of the students during the discussion?

_____

_____

_____

_____

_____

- What were the characteristics and behaviors of the instructor during the discussion?

- What were the results of the discussion? (List as many ideas as you can.)

TAKE IT TO THE CLASSROOM ACTIVITIES

Take It to the Classroom activities are designed to support you in applying the module's concepts to the classroom. Course objectives will be met most effectively and learning will be most beneficial if the activities are completed in conjunction with the material found in the online course.

Several methods can be used to stimulate effective discussions in the classroom. Consider incorporating some of the following methods into your class to encourage discussion.

Brainstorming

Brainstorming has the goal of developing as many responses, solutions, and ideas as possible. The key to brainstorming is to avoid judgment until after all ideas have been listed. Quantity of ideas matters more than quality. Sometimes, outrageous ideas spark realistic actions.

Notes for Planning This Activity:

SWOT Analysis

SWOT means Strengths, Weaknesses, Opportunities, and Threats. Careful consideration of these areas helps to thoroughly analyze an idea or solution to a problem.

Notes for Planning This Activity:

Model Development

This discussion strategy asks students to develop a model or a representation of a concept, idea, or theory.

Notes for Planning This Activity:

Consensus Building

This strategy requires the entire class (or discussion group) to come to a consensus on a solution. The resulting discussion generally covers most of the important areas of the question.

Notes for Planning This Activity:

Metaphor Creation

Creation of a metaphor asks students to compare a concept they are learning to something they already understand. This strategy requires the breaking down of individual components of a concept or problem.

Notes for Planning This Activity:

See the *Idea List for Classroom Activities Worksheet* at the end of this section.

CONFLICT RESOLUTION

Summarize the importance of effective conflict resolution and explain the factors to consider when choosing a conflict resolution approach.

Summarize each of the following conflict resolution approaches and note the situation(s) in which each might be most effective.

The Authoritarian Approach

Compromise

New Solution Creation

Letting It Go

■ ■ ■ DIVERSITY CONSIDERATIONS ■ ■ ■

Conflict resolution is another area in which cultural background has a significant influence. Examples include the student whose culture teaches that it is the duty of the authority figure (the instructor) to resolve the conflict or the student whose cultural background views conflict resolution decisions as the responsibility of a specific gender. Consider how you would approach these situations (or others) in a manner that supports effective conflict resolution and respects the backgrounds of others.

DIVERSITY REFLECTIONS

- How would you approach a student whose belief system did not provide for conflict resolution as expected in Western culture?

_____

_____

_____

_____

_____

- How might you prepare this student for the Western workplace?

_____

_____

_____

_____

_____

GENERAL STRATEGIES FOR RESOLVING CONFLICT

Note general suggestions for conflict resolution and summarize each of the following guidelines for resolving conflict. You may find it helpful to create an example for each step by using a situation that you have encountered in the past. Consider whether the outcome might have been different if you had used the suggested steps.

Evaluate the Situation

Know Your Goal

Choose Your Approach

Maintain Professionalism

Offer an Explanation

Evaluate the Outcome

USING ACTIVE LEARNING TECHNIQUES

Summarize the benefits of active learning to adult learners. Then, summarize each of the components of active learning listed below and give an example of each based on your current course content.

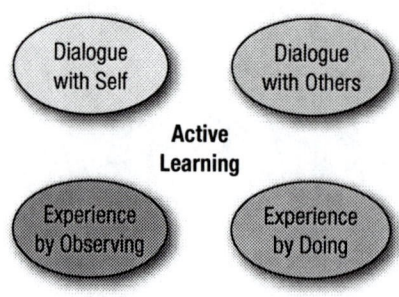

Components of Active Learning

Dialogue with Self

Dialogue with Others

Experience by Observing

Experience by Doing

GENERAL STRATEGIES FOR USING ACTIVE LEARNING TECHNIQUES

Summarize the benefits of each of the following strategies for using active learning techniques. Use specific examples from your courses whenever possible.

Consider Individual Activities

Implement Group Activities

Use Experiential Activities

Use Writing and Presenting as an Active Learning Tool

Encourage Learners to Think

TAKE IT
TO THE CLASSROOM
ACTIVITIES

Take It to the Classroom activities are designed to support you in applying the module's concepts to the classroom. Course objectives will be met most effectively and learning will be most beneficial if the activities are completed in conjunction with the material found in the online course.

Consider variations of the following activities as active learning tools for your courses. Adjust them as needed to meet the needs of your class and students.

Issue Paper

Ask students to write about both sides of an issue related to your course.

Notes for Planning This Activity:

Muddiest Point

Ask students to write about the muddiest (or least clear) point about a concept, lecture, or section of your course. This allows them to verbalize their areas of confusion and allows you to see exactly where students are missing the point.

Notes for Planning This Activity:

The Learning Journal

Ask students to keep an ongoing learning journal about their process of learning and studying, about their insights related to the topics, about their confusions, or any other focus you want. Students will learn as they reflect on their learning.

Notes for Planning This Activity:

Pre-Topic Writing

Ask students to write everything they know about a topic prior to diving into the topic in reading and lecture. This strategy encourages students to focus on what they know and develop questions that should be answered during your lecture. With this preliminary work, they are likely to pay more attention to the material as you are presenting it and as they are reading it in their textbooks.

Notes for Planning This Activity:

Student-Generated Test Questions

Ask students to develop potential test questions (and corresponding answers with a justification) as they go through the reading, complete an activity, or review their lecture notes. This process will help them organize the content, determine the important points, and study for the answers.

Notes for Planning This Activity:

End-of-Class Summary

Ask students to write a one-page summary of each lecture and submit it to you for your review. This will force students to pay attention, organize the lecture, determine what they know and do not know, and practice concise writing. Alternatively, ask them to trade papers with their classmates and review each others' summaries. The classmates can revise the summaries as they see fit.

Notes for Planning This Activity:

Poster Presentation

Ask students to develop a poster presentation about a specific topic within your course content. Many students are fearful of speaking in public. By starting off with a poster presentation, students may be more comfortable with the presentation format. Students may respond more easily to informal questions about the poster than they would in a more formal presentation format. Consider looking up guidelines for poster presentations on Web sites of professional organizations related to your industry.

Notes for Planning This Activity:

Key Word Expert

At the beginning of the course (or topic area), assign each student a key word that will be discussed during the class. Instruct students to be prepared to make a very brief presentation on the key word at the appropriate point in lecture. This strategy will help to break up a lecture and provide practice in presenting.

Notes for Planning This Activity:

PowerPoint Presentation

Ask students to develop a PowerPoint presentation on a topic of the course. Again, this strategy may alleviate some of the stress associated with speaking in public by providing a kind of prop for students. You can ask students to present and discuss each slide, or the PowerPoint slides can serve as a stand-alone presentation similar to a poster presentation where viewers ask questions.

Notes for Planning This Activity:

Student Teaching

Ask students to teach a portion of the content to small groups or to the entire class. When students are required to teach information, they must know the information at a higher level.

Notes for Planning This Activity:

See the *Idea List for Classroom Activities Worksheet* at the end of this section.

REFLECTION QUESTIONS

Be sure to record your answers to these questions in the space provided and file them in the appropriate section of your Professional Development Portfolio.

- What other writing activities could you use to help students learn the material and practice their writing skills?

  _____

  _____

  _____

  _____

  _____

- What other hands-on activities could you use to help students master course content?

  _____

  _____

  _____

  _____

  _____

- In what situations does a student's ability to think critically and creatively impact the situation significantly? (Make a list of specific situations to share as examples with your students. Keep adding to the list throughout the course.)

  _____

  _____

  _____

  _____

  _____

- What specific thinking skills will your students need in their field?

  _____

  _____

  _____

  _____

- How might you help students develop these skills within the context of your course?

  _____

  _____

  _____

  _____

LEARNING ACTIVITIES

The following activities are designed to support you in applying the module concepts to your teaching activities. Use the "Notes for Planning This Activity" spaces to record your ideas and to note resources. Complete each activity and submit as directed by your campus faculty development director. File copies of your activities and any evaluation comments you receive in your Professional Development Portfolio.

Active Learning Assignment

Develop an active learning experience for your students for each major topic on your course outline. Vary the experiences between individual, group, and experiential and include both writing and presentation activities. If you wish, use the Idea List of Classroom Activities worksheet (at the end of this section) as a starting point. Be sure to add your ideas to this list for future courses.

Notes for Planning This Activity:

Keeping Students Engaged

Work with several colleagues who teach in your program to brainstorm attention-capturing and engaging activities for your courses. First make a list of major topic areas you teach; then brainstorm ideas for each topic area. Brainstorming means that individuals take turns throwing out as many ideas as they can without judging the value or feasibility of the ideas. The purpose is to come up with as many ideas as possible and to leave the judgment of those ideas for later. Use this idea list to generate activities for your own class to keep and maintain student attention. Engaging activities do not have to be major productions. Even small activities can significantly keep your students' attention.

Notes for Planning This Activity:

Critical-Thinking Research

Search the Internet for information on teaching critical thinking to college students. Select some of the information that interests you and will help your students. Incorporate mini-lectures on critical-thinking topics in your course. See if you can teach students a topic and then immediately implement the concept in a discussion or activity.

Notes for Planning This Activity:

LEARNING OBJECTIVES REVISITED

Review the Learning Objectives for Section 3 and rate your level of achievement for each objective using the rating scale provided. Following your assessment, determine the steps you need to take to meet the objective effectively. For each objective on which you do not rate yourself as a 3, outline a plan of action that you will take to achieve the objective fully. Include a time frame for this plan. Review completed Learning Activities for specific areas in which you need further development. Include the assessment and goals that you write in your Professional Development Portfolio. You may wish to use the Instructor Improvement Plan to set goals to further work toward learning objectives.

1 = did not successfully achieve objective
2 = understand what is needed, but need more study or practice
3 = achieved learning objective thoroughly

	1	2	3
13. The instructor will be able to develop an effective and interesting lecture appropriate for a specific learner population.	☐	☐	☐
14. The instructor will identify effective listening skills and evaluate his or her own skills related to listening to students.	☐	☐	☐
15. The instructor will identify effective questioning techniques and positive ways to field student questions.	☐	☐	☐
16. The instructor will identify skills needed to facilitate effective discussions in the classroom, both in large and small group situations.	☐	☐	☐
17. The instructor will be able to explain the importance of active learning in the classroom and demonstrate the ability to develop these types of activities for class.	☐	☐	☐

STEPS TO ACHIEVE UNMET OBJECTIVES

Steps	Date
1. _____	_____
2. _____	_____
3. _____	_____
4. _____	_____

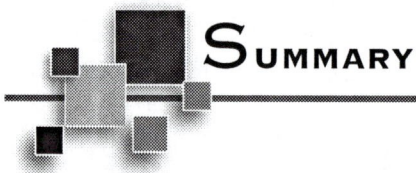

SUMMARY

Section 3 discussed the specific tasks and associated skills required in conducting an effective class. Areas of instruction included making excellent presentations and planning effective lectures. The section also gave discussion and questioning strategies for engaging learners in lecture and activity situations. Finally, Section 3 discussed the importance of active learning for the adult learner and provided a few ideas on how to incorporate active learning experiences into the classroom. This section provides only a small amount of the information that an excellent instructor requires, but should give the instructor solid foundational skills and help establish areas of strength and weakness and opportunities for further improvement.

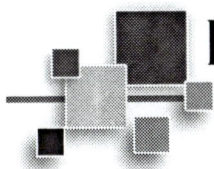

INSTRUCTOR IMPROVEMENT PLAN

Complete the Instructor Improvement Plan for Section 3 at this time. Take the necessary time to prepare a thoughtful, detailed improvement plan. Complete the form and keep it available as you plan and teach your classes for the next few terms. Note your progress, problems, successes, and questions over the next three to six months. At that time, reevaluate the plan and set new goals. Depending on the format you have selected for your Professional Development Portfolio, file the elements of your instructional plan in the appropriate sections. Record the dates for reassessing your goals on the professional development schedule at the beginning of your portfolio.

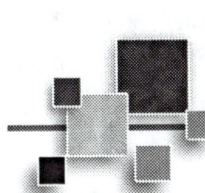

PROFESSIONAL DEVELOPMENT PORTFOLIO ELEMENTS

To finish Section 3, insert your completed responses, reflections, and activities from the section into the designated parts of your Professional Development Portfolio.

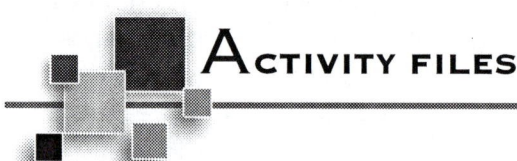

ACTIVITY FILES

The activities on the following pages will help you achieve the Section 3 learning objectives that are referenced throughout the section. In the online module, there are links to PDF files with supporting documents or worksheets for these activities.

INSTRUCTOR CHARACTERISTICS RATING SHEET

Rate yourself in the following areas using the scale of 1 to 5. Also make comments that will help in improvement, and identify specific actions you might take to improve. Be honest. Everyone can make improvements. Excellent instructors understand this and are always seeking areas they can improve.

1 = Poor; need significant improvement
2 = Fair; need some improvement
3 = Good; can improve slightly
4 = Great; very little improvement required
5 = Excellent; serve as a valuable role model for students

CHARACTERISTICS	1	2	3	4	5	COMMENTS AND STRATEGIES FOR IMPROVEMENT
1. Demonstration of respect for students						
2. Lack of arrogance with respect to teaching position, educational achievements, or career success						
3. Enthusiasm about industry						
4. Enthusiasm about course and content						
5. Support of institution in which you are teaching						
6. Support of textbook						
7. Attitude toward students' abilities to succeed in their careers						
8. Attitude toward students' abilities to learn						
9. Attitude toward students in general						
10. Willingness to take constructive criticism and use for improvement						

CHARACTERISTICS	1	2	3	4	5	COMMENTS AND STRATEGIES FOR IMPROVEMENT
11. Ability to foster open communication in the classroom						
12. Ability to develop a good rapport with students						
13. Ability to create a safe learning environment						
14. Willingness to help students outside of class						
15. Empathy toward challenges of the adult learner						
16. Understanding of the adult learner						
17. Knowledge of students in your class						
18. Ability to facilitate creative, interesting, and active discussion						
19. Ability to ask thought-provoking questions						
20. Ability to field student questions so that students will continue to ask questions and gain knowledge from your answers						
21. Willingness to acknowledge success, experiences, and current knowledge of individual students in your class						
22. Willingness to admit when you make a mistake						
23. Willingness to admit when you do not know something						
24. Willingness to do what it takes to help each student succeed						
25. Willingness to continue to improve in your teaching abilities						

IDEA LIST FOR CLASSROOM ACTIVITIES

 Use the following idea list to implement active learning and engaging discussions in your class and to spark additional ideas. Write down your ideas for additional activities so you do not forget them.

Discussion Strategies

❑ **Brainstorming.** Brainstorming has the goal of developing as many responses, solutions, and ideas as possible. The key to brainstorming is to avoid judgment until after all ideas have been listed. Quantity of ideas matters more than quality. Sometimes, outrageous ideas spark realistic ideas.

❑ **SWOT Analysis.** SWOT means Strengths, Weaknesses, Opportunities, and Threats. Careful consideration of these areas helps to thoroughly analyze an idea or solution to a problem.

❑ **Model Development.** This discussion strategy asks students to develop a model or a representation of a concept, idea, or theory.

❑ **Consensus Building.** This strategy requires that the entire class (or discussion group) come to a consensus on a solution. The resulting discussion generally covers most of the important areas of the question.

❑ **Metaphor Creation.** Creation of a metaphor asks students to compare a concept they are learning to something they already understand. This strategy requires the breaking down of individual components of a concept or problem.

❑ **Developing an Analogy.** The instructor asks students to develop an analogy for a difficult concept. For example, how is the medical office like a garden? Students should come up with weeds (office whiners who stifle productivity), gardener (office manager), fertilizer (positive feedback or training), etc. The point is to get students to think about details of a situation, concept, environment, etc. This works well as an in-class discussion.

❑ **The Bad Example.** The instructor asks students to write a bad example of a concept. Often students learn best from the bad example rather than the ideal.

❑ **Application Cards.** Instructors ask students to write down a listing of applications as they think of them during a teaching session. Students should aim to answer the question, "How will you use this in your workplace?" Instructors can discuss various responses as a class group at end of session.

❑ **Concept Map.** Instructors ask students to develop a concept map for a concept. This works well for medical procedures, organ systems, etc. The topic is placed in the center of a paper and lines are drawn to different aspects of the topic. For example, in the topic, "drawing blood," lines are drawn to safety procedures list, patient education list, blood draw procedures, set-up procedures, equipment and supplies, clean-up procedures, what could go wrong list, etc.

❑ **The Categorization Grid.** Instructors ask students to develop a categorization grid and complete it during a lecture or as a group project. For example, for A&P, the categories might be anatomy, physiological processes, diseases and disorders, s/s, treatment, prevention, drugs, etc.

❑ **Flowchart.** Instructors ask students to develop a flowchart for a procedure. For example, develop a flowchart for setting up and conducting an EKG procedure. What do students do first, second, third, etc.? This is good preparation for a lab activity.

Active Learning Experiences

- ❏ **Issue Paper.** Ask students to write about both sides of an issue related to your course.

- ❏ **Designated Sides.** As with an issue paper, ask students to write about a controversial topic, but designate which side the student is to take, regardless of personal opinion. Use these papers as starters for discussion. Designating sides frees students from being inhibited about personal views.

- ❏ **The Term Paper.** Students research a topic thoroughly over the long term. Consider assessing and perhaps providing a grade at every stage to assist students in fully developing writing skills. Stages might include: Development of Topic and Treatment of Ideas, Research of Topic, Synthesis of Information, Organization of Information, Explanation of Ideas, Analysis of Information, Writing of Paper, Submission Format.

- ❏ **Invented Dialogue.** Ask students to write the dialogue that might occur related to a topic of discussion. This activity works well in relational areas such as patient interaction, conflict negotiation, job search, and management. Ask students to write a dialogue that is effective and then one that is not effective in achieving the goals.

- ❏ **One-Sentence Summary.** Students write a summary of a lecture, reading, concept, etc., in one sentence. With practice, students learn to make every word count, to formulate effective sentences, and to summarize information well.

- ❏ **Muddiest Point.** Ask students to write about the muddiest (or least clear) point about a concept, lecture, or section of your course. This allows them to verbalize their areas of confusion and allows you to see exactly where students are missing the point.

- ❏ **Letter to the Editor.** Assign students to write a letter to the editor to refute or respond to a current article. Consider reviewing examples prior to the assignment and reviewing guidelines from local journals. Also consider using professional journal examples in addition to local newspaper and magazine examples.

- ❏ **Office Documents.** Assign students to write reports, memos, letters, or educational brochures or documents for a potential employer in their field. Consider using real-life assignments to assist local organizations.

- ❏ **Class Minutes.** Assign each student to take notes in class for a session and then to write up the minutes using standard minutes format. The minutes can then be discussed as a class, corrections can be made, and the final copy can be distributed as a study tool.

- ❏ **The Learning Journal.** Ask students to keep an ongoing learning journal about their process of learning and studying, about their insights related to the topics, about their confusions, or any other focus you want. Students will learn as they reflect on their learning.

- ❏ **Pre-Topic Writing.** Ask students to write everything they know about a topic prior to diving into the topic in reading and lecture. This strategy encourages students to focus on what they know and develop questions that should be answered during your lecture. With this preliminary work, they are likely to pay more attention to the material as you are presenting it and as they are reading it in their text.

- ❏ **Student-Generated Test Questions.** Ask students to develop potential test questions (and corresponding answers with a justification) as they go through the reading, complete an activity, or review their lecture notes. This process will help them organize the content, determine the important points, and study for the answers.

❏ **End-of-Class Summary.** Ask students to write a one-page summary of each lecture and submit it to you for your review. This will force students to pay attention, organize the lecture, determine what they know and do not know, and practice concise writing. Alternatively, ask them to trade papers with their classmates and review each others' summaries. The classmates can revise the summaries as they see fit.

❏ **Poster Presentation.** Ask students develop a poster presentation about a specific topic within your course content. Many students are very fearful of speaking in public. By starting them off with a poster presentation, students may be more comfortable with the presentation format. Students may respond more easily to informal questions about the poster than they would in a more formal presentation format. Consider looking up guidelines for poster presentations on Web sites of professional organizations related to your industry.

❏ **Key Word Expert.** At the beginning of the course (or topic area), assign each student a key word that will be discussed during the class. Instruct students to be prepared to make a very brief presentation on the key word at the appropriate point in the lecture. This strategy will help to break up a lecture and provide practice in presenting.

❏ **PowerPoint Presentation.** Ask students to develop a PowerPoint presentation on a topic of the course. Again, this strategy may alleviate some of the stress associated with speaking in public by providing a kind of prop for students. You can ask students to present and discuss each slide, or the PowerPoint slides can serve as a stand-alone presentation similar to a poster presentation where viewers ask questions.

❏ **Student Teaching.** Ask students to teach a portion of the content to small groups or to the entire class. When students must teach information, they must know the information at a higher level.

❏ **Student Demonstration.** As in the student teaching activity, ask a student or group of students to demonstrate a technique, use of a piece of equipment, or something else related to your class. Consider asking them to do this as if they were explaining the process or equipment to a client, patient, or customer. How do they make technical information understandable for these populations?

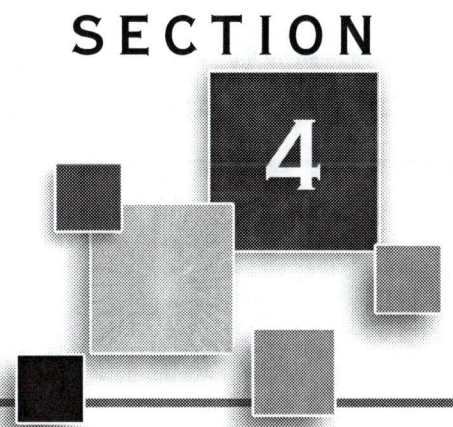

SECTION 4

GRADING AND ASSESSMENT

LEARNING OBJECTIVES

Upon successful completion of Section 4, the instructor will have achieved the following objectives. Check off each of the objectives as you have mastered it. You will have the opportunity to assess your performance on each objective at the end of Section 4.

18. The instructor will be able to identify important purposes of assessment of the adult learner.
19. The instructor will be able to identify the important characteristics of effective feedback and to conduct a self-assessment in providing feedback with the goal of establishing an improvement plan.
20. The instructor will be able to develop a variety of informal assessments for use with adult learners.
21. The instructor will be able to develop fair and equitable grading polices for a course.
22. The instructor will identify specific steps to be taken to reduce the opportunity for academic dishonesty in classes.

INTRODUCTORY QUESTIONS

- What is the purpose of grading and assessment in your class?
- How many different ways can you assess a student's progress?
- What are effective and ineffective ways to provide feedback to students?
- What are fair and equitable grading policies?
- What is included in academic dishonesty?

OVERVIEW

Section 4 provides an overview of the important considerations in assessing and grading the adult learner. It discusses the basics of test development, provides alternatives to grading for the assessment of students, and suggests guidelines for establishing grading policies and reducing opportunities for academic dishonesty in a class.

SUGGESTED GENERAL GUIDELINES: ASSESSMENT AND EVALUATION OF THE ADULT LEARNER

Compare and contrast assessment and evaluation and note the purposes of each in your classes.

GENERAL STRATEGIES FOR USING ASSESSMENT

Note how you could apply each of the assessment strategies listed below in your classes.

Assess Student Progress

Encourage Student Motivation

Obtain Feedback on the Effectiveness of Your Teaching

Determine if Students are Meeting Course Objectives

Encourage Students to Reflect on Learning Strategies

Conduct Informal Assessments

REFLECTION QUESTIONS

Be sure to record your answers to these questions in the space provided and file them in the appropriate section of your Professional Development Portfolio.

- What kind of assessments do you conduct in your course?

_____

_____

_____

_____

_____

- What specific purposes do you have for assessment in your course?

_____

_____

_____

_____

_____

- How do you use the information you gain from the assessments?

TAKE IT TO THE CLASSROOM ACTIVITIES

Take It to the Classroom activities are designed to support you in applying the module's concepts to the classroom. Course objectives will be met most effectively and learning will be most beneficial if the activities are completed in conjunction with the material found in the online course.

Many activities can be used to assess students' progress in your class. Consider the following activities (some of which you might have considered for other purposes) as quick assessment tools.

One-Minute Paper

Ask students to spend one minute writing a brief summary of a chunk of information. Alternatively, ask students to spend one minute writing all they know about a topic prior to the lecture.

Notes for Planning This Activity:

Muddiest Point

Ask students to describe the most unclear points of a concept after a lecture or after a reading assignment. This allows them to verbalize their areas of confusion and allows you to see exactly where students are missing the point. The instructor should review these points and address them in class or in the next class. This strategy is especially useful at the start of a teaching session, after a reading assignment, or after a lab or hands-on activity.

Notes for Planning This Activity:

True/False Statements

Place several true/false statements on a PowerPoint slide, a handout, or the board after a teaching session. Ask students to determine if each statement is true or false and to explain why. The class must come to a consensus, which typically fosters detailed discussion. This strategy works best with difficult concepts and subtle differences where students need a detailed understanding of the material.

Notes for Planning This Activity:

End-of-Class Summary

Asks students to summarize on one page the information from a teaching session (part or section or lab activity). The instructor can then use the information to determine the misunderstandings and discuss them during the next session as appropriate.

Notes for Planning This Activity:

Labeling on PowerPoint Assessment

Conduct a brief assessment after a teaching session using your PowerPoint slide show. Ask questions, use diagrams from image libraries, use matching lists, and so forth. This can be done without a PowerPoint slide show; however, it is very easy to incorporate assessment slides periodically into a slide show. This practice helps students get into the habit of paying attention because they know there will be a periodic assessment.

Notes for Planning This Activity:

Misconception/Preconception Check

Prior to diving into a new topic, especially a topic that has a higher level of personal or public opinion, controversy, or related issues, ask students to write down their preconceptions of the topic and related issues. What do they currently know? What do they think is myth or misconception? Where might the general public be in error about facts? What are the basic facts that they think are true? What is the source of their current information? Re-assess after new information has been provided.

Notes for Planning This Activity:

Pre-Topic Diagnostic Assessment

A diagnostic assessment prior to a topic allows students to assess for themselves what they already know, and then, after the answers are provided, determine what they do not know. This strategy will help to point out important aspects of the coming information, show students what they need to learn, and focus their attention by giving them questions that they now need to have answered. These assessments should be viewed as a help in learning, not as a threat to students.

Notes for Planning This Activity:

Assignment Assessments

In addition to assessing students on their acquisition of facts using end of topic exams, try assessing students on what they learn from assignments, either hands-on lab activities or other projects. The focus of the assessment can be background information and how it is used to achieve the goals of the assignment. If assignments have well-defined objectives, the assignment assessment can help to validate that students have achieved the objectives. Assignment assessments can also help to focus students' attention on the details of the assignment since they know they will be tested on their knowledge and skill acquisition.

Notes for Planning This Activity:

Collaborative Assessments

Collaborative assessments assess student skill and knowledge acquisition and help students continue to learn the information. These collaborative groups can be pairs of students taking an assessment together or small groups of students (preferably fewer than five students) working together to find the answers to assessment questions. The more difficult or complex the questions, the more students in the group will have to collaborate to achieve the answer.

Notes for Planning This Activity:

No Penalty Quiz

No penalty quizzes serve a very useful purpose in a classroom. Students can document what they know without the stress of performing on a graded quiz. This allows students to assess for themselves where they need to put in more study time, clarify confusions, or get additional assistance. Consider giving several of these quizzes over the entire course and allowing students to pick their top four or five scores to include in their grade for the course. This strategy helps to ensure that students will take the quizzes seriously. Instructors can also grade the students' correction of the quizzes, if grades are needed.

Notes for Planning This Activity:

Written Portion of Practical Exams

In many areas, students must demonstrate achievement of practical, hands-on skills. Consider adding a written portion to this skill assessment to help students connect the theoretical portion of the skill to the skill itself. Also consider assessing how well the student connects the skill to the real-world workplace.

Notes for Planning This Activity:

Mid-Lecture Assessments

Consider providing students with a list of questions that they should address either during or after a lecture based on the lecture material. This strategy helps students to stay focused on the lecture or activity and to stay active in their learning.

Notes for Planning This Activity:

Student-Generated Exam Questions

Ask students to develop several exam questions that may be used for the next quiz or class exam. Students' questions are often much more difficult than the instructor's questions. They should also develop a key (answer sheet) with textbook or other references to validate their answers. Also consider asking them to develop feedback for each alternative answer, whether the answer is correct or incorrect. (For example, they should explain why a response in a multiple choice is incorrect.) Encourage complex questions, use of Bloom's taxonomy to develop higher-order questions, and creativity. Instructors can use these questions to determine if the students understand the material being presented at the appropriate depth.

Notes for Planning This Activity:

REFLECTION QUESTIONS

Be sure to record your answers to these questions in the space provided and file them in the appropriate section of your Professional Development Portfolio.

- How do you currently conduct informal assessments during your class or hands-on activities? (List all the ways you do this.)

_____

_____

_____

_____

_____

- How can you increase the assessment of your students? (List techniques that would be appropriate for your classes.)

_____

_____

_____

_____

_____

PROVIDING EFFECTIVE FEEDBACK

State the importance of providing feedback to students and summarize each of the goals for providing feedback.

GENERAL STRATEGIES FOR PROVIDING FEEDBACK

Summarize the following strategies for providing feedback and give an example of how each could be applied in your classes.

Describe Behavior

Give Feedback That Is Supportive, Not Punitive

Give Feedback That Is Specific

Consider Timing

Show Empathy

Make an Action Plan Based on Feedback

Follow Up With the Student

See the *Feedback Assessment Checklist* at the end of this section.

REFLECTION QUESTIONS

Be sure to record your answers to these questions in the space provided and file them in the appropriate section of your Professional Development Portfolio.

- How often do you provide feedback to your students? In what form?

_____

_____

_____

_____

_____

- Do you often write comments on assignments or quizzes, or do you let a grade stand on its own?

_____

_____

_____

_____

_____

- How often do you provide verbal feedback to students? How do students respond?

_____

_____

_____

_____

_____

BUILDING ASSESSMENT TOOLS

Summarize the importance of effective assessment in the classroom. Then, summarize each of the following considerations pertaining to assessment and note how each can be applied in your classes.

Match Assessment to Course Objectives

See *Bloom's Taxonomy Word List* at the end of this section.

Assess Learning at Different Stages of Bloom's Taxonomy

Assess Knowledge

Note when assessment at the *knowledge* level is appropriate.

```
┌─────────────────────────────────────────────────────────────┐
│                                                             │
│                                                             │
│                                                             │
│                                                             │
│                                                             │
│                                                             │
│                                                             │
└─────────────────────────────────────────────────────────────┘
```

TAKE IT
TO THE CLASSROOM
ACTIVITIES (KNOWLEDGE)

Take It to the Classroom activities are designed to support you in applying the module's concepts to the classroom. Course objectives will be met most effectively and learning will be most beneficial if the activities are completed in conjunction with the material found in the online course.

For each of the following suggested strategies for assessing knowledge, write an example that could be used in your courses.

- Ask questions that are answered with factual information.

Notes for Planning This Activity:

- Use multiple choice, matching, and true/false questions.

Notes for Planning This Activity:

- Ask students to identify appropriate tools, techniques, or procedures for a certain task in your field.

Notes for Planning This Activity:

- At different stations (as in a lab exam), have students label items or parts of equipment that are specific to your field.

Notes for Planning This Activity:

- Ask students to reproduce a design, table, chart, or other summary of information.

Notes for Planning This Activity:

- Have students match required materials to a process in your field.

Notes for Planning This Activity:

- Ask students to recite or reproduce policies, procedures, or codes that are foundational to your field.

Notes for Planning This Activity:

Assess Comprehension

Note when assessment at the *comprehension* level is appropriate.

TAKE IT
TO THE CLASSROOM
ACTIVITIES (COMPREHENSION)

For each of the following suggested strategies for assessing comprehension, write an example that could be used in your courses.

- On tests, use short answer items that ask students to describe or explain an event, summarize a main idea, interpret a meaning, paraphrase, or give examples.

Notes for Planning This Activity:

- Provide students with a scenario from a movie, role play, story, or other media and ask them to interpret its meaning as it relates to the topic of study.

Notes for Planning This Activity:

- Provide students with a situation and ask them to explain why the events occurred as they did.

Notes for Planning This Activity:

- Select ideas and quotations from your field and ask students to rephrase them in their own words.

Notes for Planning This Activity:

- Ask students to explain a process, procedure, or other phenomenon.

Notes for Planning This Activity:

Assess Application

Note when assessment at the *application* level is appropriate.

TAKE IT TO THE **CLASSROOM** ACTIVITIES

For each of the following suggested strategies for assessing application, write an example that could be used in your courses.

- On written tests, ask questions in a way that requires students to actively manipulate information.

Notes for Planning This Activity:

- Use problem sets that require formulas and computations.

Notes for Planning This Activity:

- Provide students with a problem or situation and ask them to locate resources that would offer information relevant to solving the problem.

Notes for Planning This Activity:

- Ask students to demonstrate a technique, such as a clinical treatment, or the use of a piece of equipment, such as computer software.

Notes for Planning This Activity:

- Have students write a report, documentation, or complete other paperwork according to the standards of your field.

Notes for Planning This Activity:

- Have students demonstrate the use of resources in your field, such as electronic media, journals, texts, or other material.

Notes for Planning This Activity:

- Evaluate students in preparing the environment for a patient, customer, or client by gathering necessary supplies, information, and other materials.

Notes for Planning This Activity:

Assess Analysis

Note when assessment at the *analysis* level is appropriate.

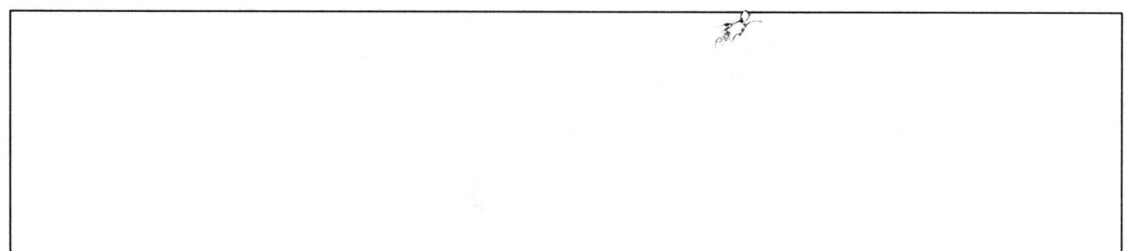

For each of the following suggested strategies for assessing analysis, write an example that could be used in your courses.

- On written tests, use essay questions that require students to examine the ideas that build a concept or contribute to an event.

Notes for Planning This Activity:

- Ask students to sort out the incidents that led to an event, to determine the ideas that led to a concept or invention, or to distinguish assumptions from fact.

Notes for Planning This Activity:

- If multiple-choice questions are used, the student should be required to make the same types of distinctions to arrive at the answer.

Notes for Planning This Activity:

- Ask students to read an article depicting a controversial topic in your field and then write an analysis of its assumptions and facts.

Notes for Planning This Activity:

- Use case studies to provide students with an issue or problem that may be encountered in your field and ask students to identify the relevant considerations in addressing the concern.

Notes for Planning This Activity:

- Provide students with a problem and ask them to identify possible causes.

Notes for Planning This Activity:

- Ask students to illustrate a concept and its component parts by completing a flowchart or concept map.

Notes for Planning This Activity:

- Hold a debate that requires students to analyze an issue from different perspectives.

Notes for Planning This Activity:

Assess Synthesis

Note when assessment at the *synthesis* level is appropriate.

```
┌─────────────────────────────────────────────────────────────────┐
│                                                                 │
│                                                                 │
│                                                                 │
│                                                                 │
│                                                                 │
└─────────────────────────────────────────────────────────────────┘
```

TAKE IT
TO THE CLASSROOM
ACTIVITIES (SYNTHESIS)

For each of the following suggested strategies for assessing synthesis, write an example that could be used in your courses.

- If written tests are the preferred method of evaluation, essay questions are the best choice for evaluating at the synthesis level. They should require students to compile information into a logical plan.

Notes for Planning This Activity:

- Ask students to develop solutions for dilemmas or problems that are likely to occur in your field.

Notes for Planning This Activity:

- Have students develop a program that would meet a need in your field.

Notes for Planning This Activity:

- Select current issues in your field and ask students to devise a response or solution.

Notes for Planning This Activity:

- Ask students to design a piece of equipment or material to meet a specific need in your field.

Notes for Planning This Activity:

- Pose several theories from your field to students and ask them to integrate relevant aspects of the theories to address a question or solve a problem.

Notes for Planning This Activity:

Assess Evaluation

Note when assessment at the *evaluation* level is appropriate.

TAKE IT
TO THE CLASSROOM
ACTIVITIES (EVALUATION)

For each of the following suggested strategies for assessing evaluation, write an example that could be used in your courses.

- Written exams at this level must require students to propose a solution or program relative to a stated need or situation.

Notes for Planning This Activity:

- Ask students to justify a proposal based on quantifiable data.

Notes for Planning This Activity:

- Ask students to articulate advantages and limitations of a solution.

Notes for Planning This Activity:

- Select a current event or issue in your field and require students to evaluate it from several perspectives, noting the advantages and limitations of each.

Notes for Planning This Activity:

- Assign a research paper that is directed at an in-depth analysis of a theory, technique, or process in your field.

Notes for Planning This Activity:

- Ask students to critique research projects or studies and make recommendations for further study.

Notes for Planning This Activity:

- Ask students to anticipate possible results and consequences of their recommendations.

Notes for Planning This Activity:

- Ask students to perform an analysis of a policy, procedure, or administrative document in your field.

Notes for Planning This Activity:

- Ask students to propose suggestions for improvement of a specific topic or situation.

Notes for Planning This Activity:

- Present students with a proposal or idea that is currently gaining popularity in your field and ask students to evaluate the proposal or idea in terms of its possible consequences and ways it might impact your field. This is especially effective with proposed legislation or regulatory actions.

Notes for Planning This Activity:

REFLECTION QUESTIONS

Be sure to record your answers to these questions in the space provided and file them in the appropriate section of your Professional Development Portfolio.

- Review the learning objectives for your course and your assessments. Do your assessments reflect the appropriate cognitive learning level as described by your objectives?

_____

_____

_____

_____

_____

GRADING POLICIES

Comment on the significance of grades and their potential impact on students, the instructor, and the institution.

GENERAL STRATEGIES FOR ESTABLISHING EQUITABLE AND FAIR GRADING POLICIES

Summarize the following considerations for establishing grading policies. Note ideas for incorporating each suggestion into your classroom protocol.

Follow the Grading Policies of Your Institution

Ensure That You are Grading What You are Supposed to Be Grading

Ensure That the Meaning of the Grade Is Appropriate

Grade to a Standard

Provide Sufficient Opportunities for Success

Determine in Advance How You Will Treat Borderline Grades

Determine in Advance How You Will Treat Makeup Work, Late Submissions, and Incomplete Work

Reducing Grade-Related Complaints

Summarize the "truth" about grade-related complaints.

```




```

GENERAL STRATEGIES FOR REDUCING GRADE-RELATED COMPLAINTS

Summarize the following strategies for reducing grade-related complaints. Note methods for incorporating each strategy into your classroom protocols.

Publicize the Grading Criteria for Each Assignment and Your Course Grading System

Make Constructive Comments to Students as You Grade Their Assignments

Keep Accurate and Current Records

Create Objective Assessment Tools

Grade and Return Assignments in a Timely Fashion

Keep Grades Confidential

Mediate Grade Disputes Effectively

PROMOTING ACADEMIC INTEGRITY

Summarize the concerns related to cheating and its effect on the class.

GENERAL STRATEGIES FOR PROMOTING ACADEMIC INTEGRITY

Using the following guidelines, record ideas for incorporating strategies for promoting academic integrity in your classroom.

Create a Culture of Integrity

Ask Students to Create an Integrity Policy

Openly Discuss Academic Integrity

Reduce the Opportunity for Cheating

Consider Using Plagiarism-Detecting Software

Secure Your Exams

Take Proactive Measures

REFLECTION QUESTIONS

Be sure to record your answers to these questions in the space provided and file them in the appropriate section of your Professional Development Portfolio.

- What specific areas of your course might be a good opportunity for academic dishonesty?

_____

_____

_____

_____

_____

- What can you do to help dissuade students from cheating?

_____

_____

_____

_____

_____

- What are the academic dishonesty policies and statements for your institution?

_____

_____

_____

_____

_____

LEARNING ACTIVITIES

The following activities are designed to support you in applying the module concepts to your teaching activities. Use the "Notes for Planning This Activity" spaces to record your ideas and to note resources. Complete each activity and submit as directed by your campus faculty development director. File copies of your activities and any evaluation comments you receive in your Professional Development Portfolio.

Grading Policies

Acquire the grading policies established for your institution. Then, develop the grading policies for your course. If the grading policies for your course have already been developed, compare them with the institutional policies. Address the following questions: How will you handle late assignments? How will you handle makeup work? How will you handle work that is submitted but is incomplete? How will you handle plagiarism? How will you handle academic dishonesty? How will you handle borderline grades? What steps will you take in a grade dispute?

Write up your policies and consider discussing them with your supervisor or an administrator at your institution. Be sure that your course policies do not conflict with your institutional policies.

Notes for Planning This Activity:

Course Assessment Brainstorming

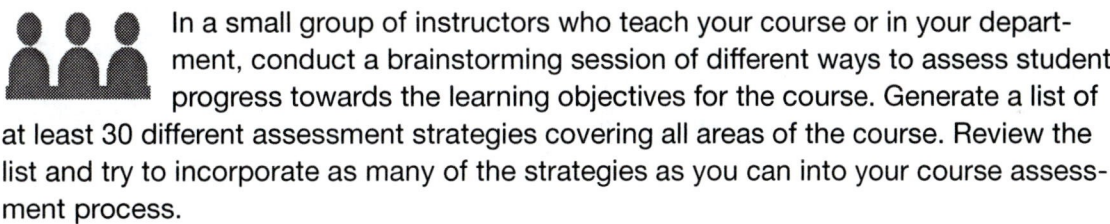 In a small group of instructors who teach your course or in your department, conduct a brainstorming session of different ways to assess student progress towards the learning objectives for the course. Generate a list of at least 30 different assessment strategies covering all areas of the course. Review the list and try to incorporate as many of the strategies as you can into your course assessment process.

Notes for Planning This Activity:

Plagiarism Software Research

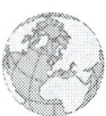 Conduct an Internet search for plagiarism software and choose two or three programs to explore in more detail. Download a trial version, if possible, and try it out for yourself. Determine the value of using this software in your course.

Notes for Planning This Activity:

Electronic Exam Generator Research

Go to http://www.examview.com and review the features of the software. Determine the value of using the software to generate exams and quizzes for your course. If possible, acquire a trial version and explore its functionality. Explore other electronic exam generator software by searching the Internet. Compare and contrast the different applications.

Notes for Planning This Activity:

LEARNING OBJECTIVES REVISITED

Review the Learning Objectives for Section 4 and rate your level of achievement for each objective using the rating scale provided. Following your assessment, determine the steps you need to take to meet the objective effectively. For each objective on which you do not rate yourself as a 3, outline a plan of action that you will take to achieve the objective fully. Include a time frame for this plan. Review completed Learning Activities for specific areas in which you need further development. Include the assessment and goals that you write in your Professional Development Portfolio. You may wish to use the Instructor Improvement Plan to set goals to further work toward learning objectives.

1 = did not successfully achieve objective
2 = understand what is needed, but need more study or practice
3 = achieved learning objective thoroughly

	1	2	3
18. The instructor will be able to identify important purposes of assessment of the adult learner.	☐	☐	☐
19. The instructor will be able to identify the important characteristics of effective feedback and to conduct a self-assessment in providing feedback with the goal of establishing an improvement plan.	☐	☐	☐
20. The instructor will be able to develop a variety of informal assessments for use with adult learners.	☐	☐	☐
21. The instructor will be able to develop fair and equitable grading polices for a course.	☐	☐	☐
22. The instructor will identify specific steps to be taken to reduce the opportunity for academic dishonesty in classes.	☐	☐	☐

STEPS TO ACHIEVE UNMET OBJECTIVES

Steps	Date
1. _____	_____
2. _____	_____
3. _____	_____
4. _____	_____

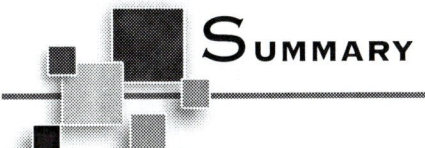

SUMMARY

Section 4 discussed the importance of assessment and grading in an academic course and the instructor's role and responsibility in this area. Different ways of evaluating student progress were highlighted in light of the various purposes and types of assessment. Section 4 also discussed how to build assessment tools appropriate for the different levels of cognitive learning. Finally, considerations were proposed for grading polices for courses and for reducing academic dishonesty. You should now be able to establish assessment and grading policies that are fair and appropriate for the needs of adult learners.

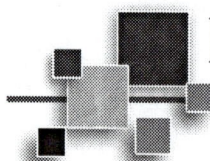

INSTRUCTOR IMPROVEMENT PLAN

Complete the Instructor Improvement Plan for Section 4 at this time. Take the necessary time to prepare a thoughtful, detailed improvement plan. Complete the form and keep it available as you plan and teach your classes for the next few terms. Note your progress, problems, successes, and questions over the next three to six months. At that time, reevaluate the plan and set new goals. Depending on the format you have selected for your Professional Development Portfolio, file the elements of your instructional plan in the appropriate sections. Record the dates for reassessing your goals on the professional development schedule at the beginning of your portfolio.

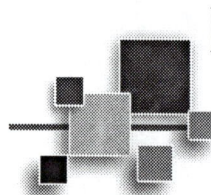

PROFESSIONAL DEVELOPMENT PORTFOLIO ELEMENTS

To finish Section 4, insert your completed responses, reflections, and activities from the section into the designated parts of your Professional Development Portfolio.

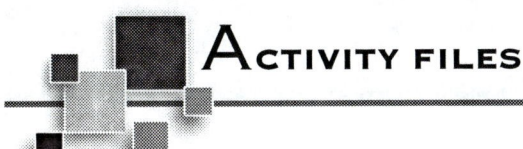

ACTIVITY FILES

The activities on the following pages will help you achieve the Section 4 learning objectives that are referenced throughout the section. In the online module, there are links to PDF files with supporting documents or worksheets for these activities.

FEEDBACK ASSESSMENT CHECKLIST

Use the following checklist and rating scale to help you improve your feedback to students. After each class session, go through the checklist and rate yourself on how well you gave feedback to your students that day. Complete this assessment for several sessions and determine if you are improving with your self-evaluation. Think about specific strategies you can use to progress.

ELEMENT OF FEEDBACK	1	2	3	4	5	COMMENTS AND IDEAS FOR IMPROVEMENT
Personal Assumptions Your assumptions about the student and student's behavior were not biased. You observed and listened carefully. You have all the information, and the information is accurate.						
Clear Expectations Your instructions and expectations were clear to yourself and your students. If needed, your expectations were in writing. You reviewed instructions and expectations with students. You are using these same expectations as a basis for your feedback.						
Motives You evaluated your motives for providing the feedback to your students. Your motive was to help students achieve their goals and not to show off, punish or embarrass students, win a disagreement, or some other motive.						
Focus of Feedback The focus of the feedback was on the behaviors of the students and their implications and not on the students themselves. You verbalized this focus in your feedback, and it was clear to students.						

ELEMENT OF FEEDBACK	1	2	3	4	5	COMMENTS AND IDEAS FOR IMPROVEMENT
Respect for Students You demonstrated that you highly respect students, even when their behavior was not appropriate. You maintained a professional demeanor, spoke calmly, listened attentively, and tried to understand the students' perspectives. You treated your students as customers.						
Feedback Statements You used "I" statements rather than "you" statements and tried to communicate your perception rather than absolute facts that you may have misinterpreted. You gave students permission to express their points of view. You made an acceptable case for your expectations.						
Intensity of Feedback You did not exaggerate, minimize, or use sarcasm. This was reflected in your word choices in that you avoided "you never," "you always," "this is the worst I have seen," and so forth.						
Directness You were direct with your statements rather than elusive. You avoided words like "maybe," "kind of," "sort of," and "I guess."						
Questions You asked questions to determine where students were having difficulties, where they think they were correct, where they think they went wrong, and how they think they performed.						
Structure of the Feedback You started with something positive, described what you saw in both positive and negative terms and areas needing improvement, and described the impact of both positive and negative behavior. You ended with a positive statement.						

ELEMENT OF FEEDBACK	1	2	3	4	5	COMMENTS AND IDEAS FOR IMPROVEMENT
Amount of Feedback You did not overwhelm the students with too much feedback at one time, but concentrated on a few elements of the behavior. You provided feedback in terms of what the students could use rather than everything you know.						
Assistance with Improvement You helped students find specific ways to improve instead of just pointing out the deficiencies. You allowed students to have input on this plan of action.						
Continuous Quality Improvement You demonstrated an attitude of continuous quality improvement reflecting the philosophy that there is always room for improvement, even in the best performances. You provided ideas for ongoing growth or expansion of skills for optimal career success.						
Empathy and Encouragement You expressed empathy if students appeared frustrated or showed poor self-esteem. You acknowledged the difficulty in the task or question and praised efforts. You helped students see failures or shortcomings as opportunities for growth.						
Emotions You maintained limited emotion toward students, especially if your emotions were negative. You allowed students to express their emotions, and you dealt with them professionally.						
Timing The timing of your feedback was as close as possible to the behavior in order to have the most impact.						
Documentation If appropriate, you documented your feedback to students appropriately explaining who, what, why, when, where, and providing a follow-up plan.						

BLOOM'S TAXONOMY WORD LIST

 Use the following word list to help you determine the cognitive level at which you teach and assess students. Add to the list as you think of new words that apply.

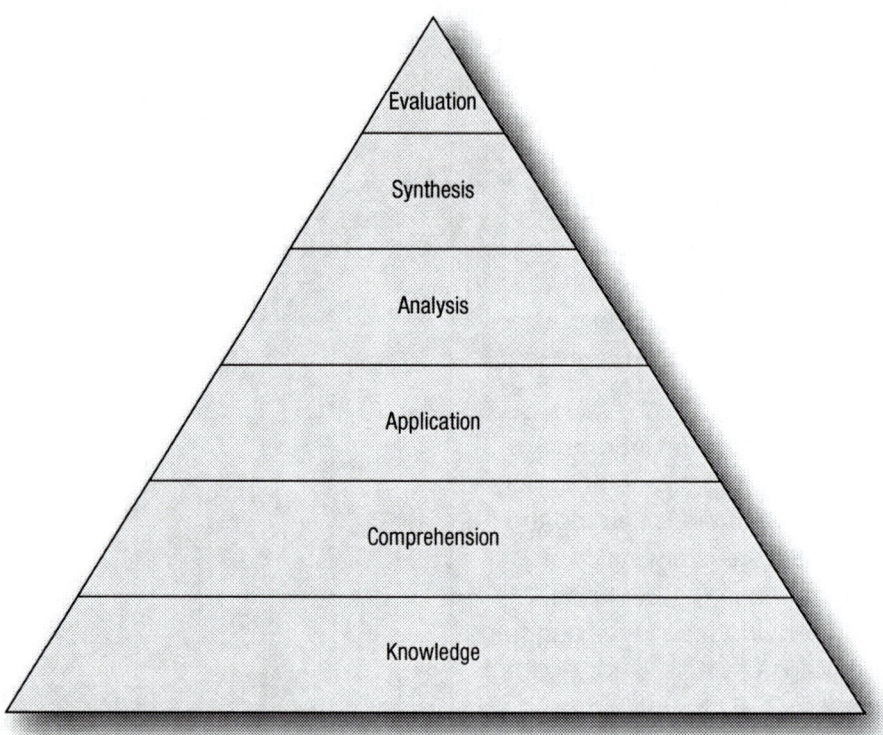

Knowledge—Observe and Recall Facts

list	define	describe	label	collect
examine	identify	tabulate	quote	name
who	when	where	how much	duplicate
arrange	memorize	recognize	relate	recall
repeat	state	reproduce	view	read
cite	count	enumerate	index	study

Comprehension—Understand Information

summarize	describe	interpret	extend	discuss
differentiate	compare	contrast	predict	associate
distinguish	estimate	classify	explain	express
indicate	locate	report	restate	review
translate	paraphrase	generalize	cite	make sense of
understand	trace	give examples	add	approximate
associate	characterize	clarify	classify	detail
elaborate	interpolate			

Application—Use Information

apply	demonstrate	calculate	complete	illustrate
show	solve	examine	modify	relate
change	classify	experiment	discover	choose
dramatize	employ	operate	interpret	practice
schedule	sketch	draw	use	write
assemble	administer	articulate	chart	act
assess	control	determine	implement	instruct
participate	preserve	prepare	teach	project
utilize	transfer	operationalize	produce	acquire
adapt	allocate	assign	attain	avoid
back up	capture	customize	derive	exercise
handle	graph	chart	manipulate	plot
price	round off	sequence	simulate	transcribe

Analysis—Organize Parts

analyze	separate	order	explain	infer
connect	classify	arrange	compare	divide
sort	appraise	criticize	categorize	differentiate
discriminate	distinguish	examine	experiment	question
test	break down	correlate	diagram	focus
illustrate	infer	limit	outline	point out
prioritize	subdivide	transform	audit	characterize
blueprint	confirm	detect	diagnose	dissect
document	file	figure out	group	investigate
lay out	maximize	minimize	proofread	query
train	size up			

Synthesis—Use Old Ideas or Facts to Create New Ideas or Facts

combine	integrate	modify	create	rearrange
substitute	plan	design	develop	invent
compose	formulate	prepare	generalize	what if
rewrite	assemble	collect	compose	construct
manage	organize	set up	prepare	propose
adapt	anticipate	collaborate	devise	express
facilitate	generate	incorporate	initiate	individualize
intervene	integrate	model	negotiate	reconstruct
reorganize	revise	validate	progress	abstract
animate	budget	code	combine	cope

(Continued)

correspond	cultivate	depict	enhance	dictate
generate	handle	import	improve	lecture
network	interface	join	overhaul	portray
prescribe	program	specify	summarize	

Evaluation—Assess Value

rank	grade	assess	evaluate	select
test	measure	recommend	convince	conclude
judge	explain	discriminate	support	defend
compare	summarize	argue	estimate	decide
predict	rate	critique	criticize	fire
interpret	justify	counsel	hire	
validate	verify			

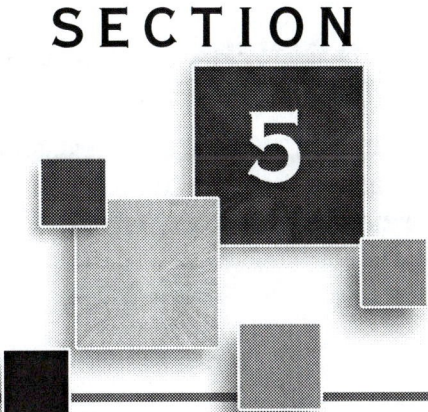

SECTION 5

EFFECTIVE CLASSROOM MANAGEMENT STRATEGIES

LEARNING OBJECTIVES

Upon successful completion of Section 5, the instructor will have achieved the following objectives. Check off each of the objectives as you have mastered it. You will have the opportunity to assess your performance on each objective at the end of Section 5.

23. The instructor will identify common strategies that will help improve student motivation.
24. The instructor will identify elements that help to create a safe learning environment for adult learners.
25. The instructor will identify common student problem situations and explain strategies to handle these situations.
26. The instructor will be able to explain why support of the institution is critical in establishing a positive learning environment and how to do this in specific areas.

INTRODUCTORY QUESTIONS

- What do you think are the top five problematic classroom situations facing instructors in the adult classroom?
- What can instructors do to prevent, minimize, or deal with these problems?
- How is the instructor's attitude contagious to students? Identify as many specific ways as you can.

OVERVIEW

Section 5 provides an overview of common, difficult classroom situations such as student inattention, nonparticipation, belligerence, and even disruptiveness, which can negatively impact the learning atmosphere. Considering the diversity of issues that can arise, this section discusses several important strategies for addressing and preventing their occurrence in order to create and maintain an environment that is conducive to learning for all the students.

SUGGESTED GENERAL GUIDELINES: SELECTING CLASSROOM MANAGEMENT STRATEGIES

Comment on the importance of the classroom environment to student success. Then, summarize each of the following guidelines for creating an effective environment. Add your own experiences to those listed in the online module.

Consider the Personal Aspects of Students

Make Course Material Meaningful

Establish a Safe Learning Environment

Confront Problem Situations Respectfully and Professionally

STUDENT MOTIVATION

List reasons for low levels of motivation in adult learners. Add others that you have recognized in your teaching or other experience.

Self-Concept

Note how self-concept can impact a student's motivation level.

GENERAL STRATEGIES FOR PROMOTING A POSITIVE SELF-CONCEPT

Note the instructor's role in influencing a student's self-concept.

What Can Instructors Do?

List actions you can take in your classroom to build positive self-concepts in your students.

What Should Instructors Not Do?

List behaviors to avoid as you build students' self-concepts.

Attitudes

Describe the elements that can influence a student's attitude toward the class.

GENERAL STRATEGIES FOR DEVELOPING POSITIVE STUDENT ATTITUDES

Summarize reasons for varying attitudes among students.

What Can Instructors Do?

List actions you can take in your classroom to develop positive student attitudes.

What Should Instructors Not Do?

List behaviors to avoid when attempting to develop positive attitudes in students.

Personal Relevance

Define personal relevance and describe its importance to the adult learners.

GENERAL STRATEGIES FOR CREATING PERSONAL RELEVANCE

Summarize the instructor's role in making course content relevant to students.

What Can Instructors Do?

Describe what an instructor can do to increase the personal relevance of course material to students.

What Should Instructors Not Do?

List those actions that reduce personal relevance of course material to students.

Tone of the Course

Define the meaning of course tone and explain the instructor's responsibility in establishing it.

```
┌─────────────────────────────────────────────────────────┐
│                                                         │
│                                                         │
│                                                         │
│                                                         │
│                                                         │
└─────────────────────────────────────────────────────────┘
```

```
┌─────────────────────────────────────────────────────────┐
│ GENERAL STRATEGIES FOR SETTING THE TONE OF THE COURSE   │
│ Consider the following suggestions for setting a        │
│ positive tone in the classroom.                         │
│                                                         │
│                                                         │
│                                                         │
│                                                         │
│                                                         │
└─────────────────────────────────────────────────────────┘
```

What Can Instructors Do?

Describe what the instructor can do to set a positive course tone.

What Should Instructors Not Do?

Describe what the instructor should avoid doing when trying to establish a positive course tone.

See the *Instructor Attitude Rating Form* at the end of this section.

REFLECTION QUESTIONS

Be sure to record your answers to these questions in the space provided and file them in the appropriate section of your Professional Development Portfolio.

- What is your personal attitude toward teaching?

_____

_____

_____

_____

_____

- What is your personal attitude toward students?

_____

_____

_____

_____

_____

- How specifically do you demonstrate your support of students?

_____

_____

_____

_____

- How specifically do you demonstrate that you love what you do as well as your industry?

_____

_____

_____

_____

_____

SAFE LEARNING ENVIRONMENTS

Describe a safe learning environment and explain what it means for students. Describe a common challenge to creating a safe learning environment.

GENERAL STRATEGIES FOR CREATING A SAFE LEARNING ENVIRONMENT

Describe each of the following strategies for establishing a safe environment. For each point, note what you can do in your classes to maximize safety. Add additional strategies that you are aware of or have used in your classes.

Set the Tone of the Course from the First Day

Evaluate Your Own Attitudes and Behaviors Toward Students, the Class, and the Industry

Teach Students Appropriate Behaviors and Explain Expectations

Create Safe Assignments and Facilitate Safe Activities

Confront Problems Immediately and Professionally

REFLECTION QUESTIONS

Be sure to record your answers to these questions in the space provided and file them in the appropriate section of your Professional Development Portfolio.

- When do you personally feel safe? (Describe the situations in detail).

_____

_____

_____

_____

_____

- In what kind of environments do you feel unsafe? (Describe the situations in detail).

_____

_____

_____

_____

- What specifically can an instructor do to create an unsafe environment?

_____

_____

_____

_____

_____

- What specifically can an instructor do to create a safe environment?

_____

_____

_____

_____

_____

PROBLEM BEHAVIORS

Summarize problem behaviors that you have encountered in the classroom and the approaches that you have used to handle them.

The Nonparticipating Student

Describe the nonparticipating student and explain possible reasons for lack of participation.

GENERAL STRATEGIES FOR WORKING WITH THE NONPARTICIPATING STUDENT

Note the important points of each of the following strategies for encouraging a student to participate.

Address the Student by Name or With Eye Contact

Use Small Groups to Lower the Risk of Participation

Talk to the Student Directly

Rearrange the Room

Use the Student's Expertise

Use Body Language

Discuss the Importance of Participation

The Know-It-All

Describe the student who "knows it all" and his or her effects on the class.

```
[blank box]
```

GENERAL STRATEGIES FOR WORKING WITH THE STUDENT WHO "KNOWS IT ALL"

Note the important points for each of the following strategies for addressing this student respectfully.

Acknowledge the Student

Challenge the Student More

Ask for Sources of Facts

Confront the Student Directly

The Rambler

Describe "the rambler" and explain the effects that this student can have on the class.

GENERAL STRATEGIES FOR WORKING WITH THE STUDENT WHO RAMBLES

Note the important points for each of the following strategies for redirecting the rambling student.

Discuss the Expectations

Refocus the Student

Write Points on the Board

The Belligerent Student

Describe behaviors frequently observed in the belligerent student.

GENERAL STRATEGIES FOR WORKING WITH THE BELLIGERENT STUDENT

Note the important points for addressing belligerent behavior that can be destructive to a safe and comfortable classroom environment.

Confront Immediately

Ask for Written Concerns

Reinforce Positive Behavior

Ask Students to Evaluate the Class Dynamics

The Complainer

Describe how complainers may appear in class and explain common reasons for complaining.

GENERAL STRATEGIES FOR WORKING WITH THE COMPLAINING STUDENT

Note strategies for addressing the complaining student and avoiding disruption to the class.

Rephrase the Complaint to Something Positive

Address the Complaints

Give Choices

Confront the Student

The Habitually Tardy Student

Describe when and how tardiness becomes a problem in a class.

GENERAL STRATEGIES FOR WORKING WITH THE HABITUALLY TARDY STUDENT

Note methods for addressing chronic tardiness.

Set Expectations

Start the Class With Important Information

Grade Attendance

Confront the Student

The Talker

Summarize the effects of side conversations, even if they are related to the class topic.

GENERAL STRATEGIES FOR WORKING WITH OVERLY TALKATIVE STUDENTS

Note important points for addressing disruptive side conversations in class.

Call On the Talkers

Wait for Them to Finish

Ask Them Not to Talk While You Are Talking

See the *Student Problem Behavior Worksheet* at the end of this section.

REFLECTION QUESTIONS

Be sure to record your answers to these questions in the space provided and file them in the appropriate section of your Professional Development Portfolio.

- What problem behaviors do you fear most as an instructor? Why?

_____

_____

_____

_____

_____

- How do you deal with these problems?

_____

_____

_____

_____

_____

SUPPORTING YOUR INSTITUTION

Describe the impact that the instructor's attitude has on students. Explain the importance of supporting the institution and its practices.

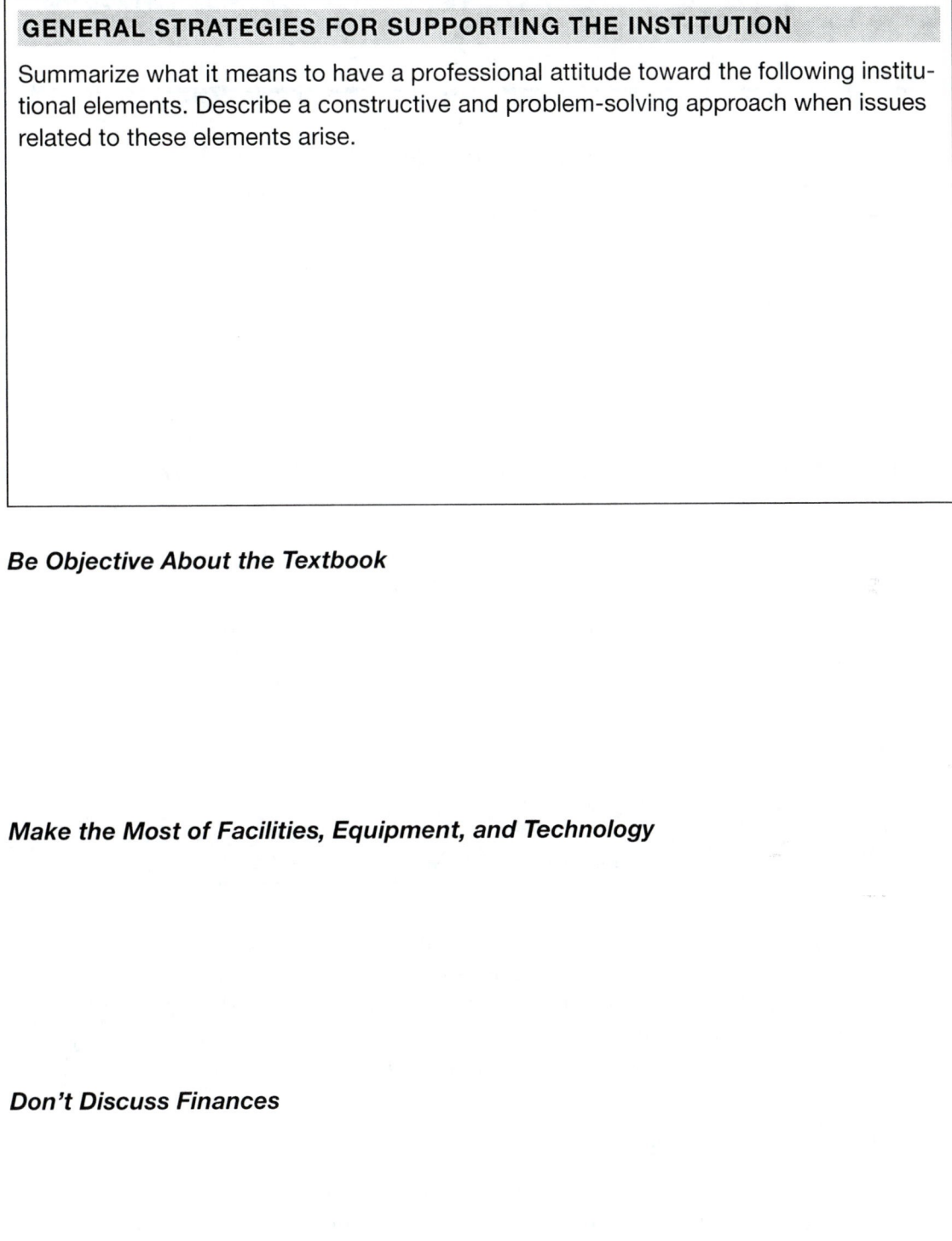

GENERAL STRATEGIES FOR SUPPORTING THE INSTITUTION

Summarize what it means to have a professional attitude toward the following institutional elements. Describe a constructive and problem-solving approach when issues related to these elements arise.

Be Objective About the Textbook

Make the Most of Facilities, Equipment, and Technology

Don't Discuss Finances

Speak Optimistically About Career Opportunities

REFLECTION QUESTIONS

Be sure to record your answers to these questions in the space provided and file them in the appropriate section of your Professional Development Portfolio.

- What frustrations do you have with your institution?

_____

_____

_____

_____

_____

- How can you positively help the institution in resolving these issues?

_____

_____

_____

_____

LEARNING ACTIVITIES

The following activities are designed to support you in applying the module concepts to your teaching activities. Use the "Notes for Planning This Activity" spaces to record your ideas and to note resources. Complete each activity and submit as directed by your campus faculty development director. File copies of your activities and any evaluation comments you receive in your Professional Development Portfolio.

Classroom Atmosphere Journal

Select one of your classes and over the course of the term (or at least several weeks), reflect on the class after each session and record your observations, impressions, and conclusions about the classroom atmosphere. Note how group dynamics, your classroom management methods, and other factors influence the tone of the class. Pay attention to the evolution of the class dynamics and make modifications to your style and techniques as needed.

Notes for Planning This Activity:

Faculty Forum

Establish a network among faculty in your department or among a group of instructors school-wide. Determine methods of communication (periodic meetings, e-mail lists, or some other method that suits your situation) to discuss issues with students and to support each other in implementing best practices in classroom management.

Notes for Planning This Activity:

Online Research for Advising Students

Conduct an online search for resources to add to your resource library. Use http://www.google.com or http://www.alltheweb.com and search using the following key words (or similar): adult classroom management, problem behaviors in the classroom, advising problem adult learners, classroom management and the adult learner, classroom management and higher education, etc.

Notes for Planning This Activity:

LEARNING OBJECTIVES REVISITED

Review the Learning Objectives for Section 5 and rate your level of achievement for each objective using the rating scale provided. Following your assessment, determine the steps you need to take to meet the objective effectively. For each objective on which you do not rate yourself as a 3, outline a plan of action that you will take to achieve the objective fully. Include a time frame for this plan. Review completed Learning Activities for specific areas in which you need further development. Include the assessment and goals that you write in your Professional Development Portfolio. You may wish to use the Instructor Improvement Plan to set goals to further work toward learning objectives.

1 = did not successfully achieve objective
2 = understand what is needed, but need more study or practice
3 = achieved learning objective thoroughly

	1	2	3
23. The instructor will identify common strategies that will help improve student motivation.	☐	☐	☐
24. The instructor will identify elements that help to create a safe learning environment for adult learners.	☐	☐	☐
25. The instructor will identify common student problem situations and explain strategies to handle these situations.	☐	☐	☐
26. The instructor will be able to explain why support of the institution is critical in establishing a positive learning environment and how to do this in specific areas.	☐	☐	☐

STEPS TO ACHIEVE UNMET OBJECTIVES

Steps	Date
1. _____	_____
2. _____	_____
3. _____	_____
4. _____	_____

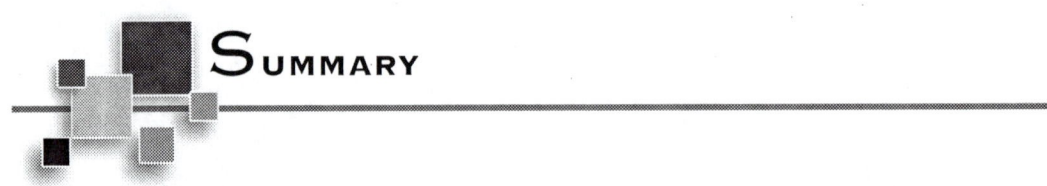

SUMMARY

Section 5 discusses four common issues related to maintaining an effective classroom. First, factors involved in student motivation are discussed along with strategies that instructors might find useful in positively influencing students to increase motivation. The characteristics of a safe learning environment are also discussed with specific actions instructors can take to ensure that students feel safe to learn and participate in the classroom. Section 5 also discusses a handful of common problem behaviors seen in classrooms with adult learners. Both positive and negative actions are discussed in light of the instructor's goal of helping learners succeed both in the course and in their chosen careers. Finally, Section 5 discusses the implications of both supporting and not supporting the institution and how it might impact the success of the instructor, student, and institution.

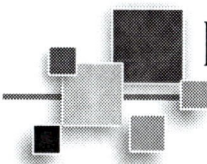

INSTRUCTOR IMPROVEMENT PLAN

Complete the Instructor Improvement Plan for Section 5 at this time. Take the necessary time to prepare a thoughtful, detailed improvement plan. Complete the form and keep it available as you plan and teach your classes for the next few terms. Note your progress, problems, successes, and questions over the next three to six months. At that time, reevaluate the plan and set new goals. Depending on the format you have selected for your Professional Development Portfolio, file the elements of your instructional plan in the appropriate sections. Record the dates for reassessing your goals on the professional development schedule at the beginning of your portfolio.

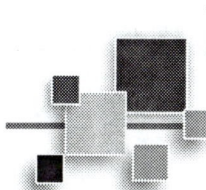

PROFESSIONAL DEVELOPMENT PORTFOLIO ELEMENTS

To finish Section 5, insert your completed responses, reflections, and activities from the section into the designated parts of your Professional Development Portfolio.

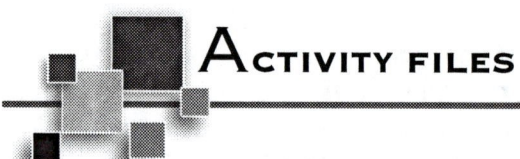

ACTIVITY FILES

The activities on the following pages will help you achieve the Section 5 learning objectives that are referenced throughout the section. In the online module, there are links to PDF files with supporting documents or worksheets for these activities.

INSTRUCTOR ATTITUDE RATING FORM

Use the following rating form to honestly evaluate your personal attitudes and the associated behaviors that you may be conveying in class. At the end of the table, add any other attitudes that you think are important in being an excellent instructor. Be very honest. When you have completed rating each item, think about ways you might be able to improve. Develop a plan to improve your attitudes if you find areas that may be a hindrance to your success in the classroom. Consider revisiting this attitude assessment form periodically throughout the course.

ATTITUDES AND ACTIONS	1	2	3	4	5	COMMENTS AND IDEAS FOR IMPROVEMENT
Praising Students You sincerely praise students at every opportunity.						
Focusing on the Positive You focus on the assets of students and the positive elements of the course, the school, the industry, the textbook, the facilities, and so forth much more than the negative.						
Encouraging Students You consciously encourage students to succeed in a specific task, to succeed in your course, and to succeed in their career.						
Assisting Students With Study Skills You consciously look for ways to help students become better students and talk to them about their study skills at every opportunity—both individually and as a class.						
Availability Outside of Class You are available to help or listen to students outside of class, and you welcome their visits.						

ATTITUDES AND ACTIONS	1	2	3	4	5	COMMENTS AND IDEAS FOR IMPROVEMENT
Starting Off Interactions With Something Positive You strive to start off every interaction with a student with a positive statement.						
Building Up Students You take every opportunity to build students up, even when they are wrong or have made mistakes.						
Focusing on Student Success Rather Than Your Own Successes You focus on the success of students rather than on your own successes or accomplishments.						
Enjoyment of Students You genuinely like students and value them as adults.						
Enjoyment of Teaching You genuinely enjoy teaching and teach because you like it rather than because you need the money.						
Respect for Students You respect students as individuals, as adults, and as future colleagues.						
Enthusiasm for Teaching You are enthusiastic about teaching and demonstrate this enthusiasm when you teach and talk with students outside of class.						
Enthusiasm for Industry You are enthusiastic about your professional industry and that of your students and demonstrate this enthusiasm when you teach and talk with students outside of class.						
Enthusiasm for Course You are enthusiastic about the course you teach and demonstrate this enthusiasm when you teach and talk with students outside of class.						

ATTITUDES AND ACTIONS	1	2	3	4	5	COMMENTS AND IDEAS FOR IMPROVEMENT
Enthusiasm for Helping Students Succeed You genuinely want to help students succeed and show this enthusiasm in all aspects of your teaching.						
Avoidance of Negativity You avoid negative comments or attitudes about all aspects of your teaching, both with your colleagues and with your students, even when there are problems.						
Support of the Institution You support the institution in all of its efforts, its policies and procedures, and its philosophies both with your colleagues and your students.						
Support of the Textbook You support the textbook, focus students' attention on the book's strong points, and use any book problems as learning opportunities, even when you think it is not the optimal book to supplement your course. Instead of criticizing the book with students, you take the appropriate channels to change the book.						
Support of the Administration You support your institution's administration in front of students and voice concerns through appropriate channels. You act to solve problems rather than complain without solutions.						
Support of Your Facilities and Equipment You support the facilities and equipment of your institution in front of students and voice concerns through appropriate channels. You act to solve problems rather than complain without solutions.						
Avoidance of Condescension Toward Students You avoid being condescending toward students at all times and maintain an attitude of support and facilitation in helping them to reach their educational and career goals.						

ATTITUDES AND ACTIONS	1	2	3	4	5	COMMENTS AND IDEAS FOR IMPROVEMENT
Demonstration of Empathy Toward Student Challenges You demonstrate an understanding and empathy toward student challenges, such as the other responsibilities they have in their lives (families, jobs, finances, and so forth). This empathy is demonstrated in your course polices, assignments, and flexibility.						
Sufficient Flexibility to Meet Student Needs You maintain sufficient flexibility within your course to meet student needs while maintaining the integrity of the course and institution.						
Maintenance of a Safe Learning Environment Your teaching environment is safe for students to participate in freely without fear of being humiliated, embarrassed, negatively confronted, or being put in other damaging situations.						
Maintenance of Control of Class You maintain control of your class at all times using effective strategies for talkers, belligerent students, ramblers, shy students, and so forth.						
Other Attitude: _____						
Other Attitude: _____						
Other Attitude: _____						

What are your top five strengths?

How do you see these strengths reflected in your classroom?

What are the five areas that you need to improve the most?

If you did improve in these areas, what impact would it have in your classroom?

STUDENT PROBLEM BEHAVIOR WORKSHEET

In a group of four or five colleagues who teach your students, complete the Student Problem Behavior Worksheet. Discuss each behavior and solution thoroughly to determine the possible causes and implications. For each problem behavior, identify the top two best responses from an instructor that will achieve the most positive results. Assume that your goal is to help students achieve success in the course, their academic endeavors, and their careers.

1. For each of the problem behaviors listed below, discuss the behavior in terms of its possible causes, how it impacts the problem student's success, and its implications for the successful classroom.
2. For each solution listed, discuss the results and how the solution will lead to meeting your goals as an instructor. Assume your goals are to ensure that all students succeed in your course, in their academic endeavors, and in their career success. Add additional solutions and additional behaviors if they are common at your institution and if time permits.
3. Finally, choose one of the solutions or design a solution as a group to meet the goals. (There may be no correct solution listed.)

Problem Behavior #1

A class includes a student who regularly tries to show the class where the instructor is wrong and criticizes the course, including homework, assignments, and assessments. This criticism expands often to the school, the textbook, and the lab facilities and equipment.

❑ **Instructor Solution A.** The instructor defends his teaching with the attitude that reflects that he is in charge of the class. When the criticism expands to the school, textbook, lab, and equipment, he agrees with the student stating that he has no control over these course elements and that he inherited them.

❑ **Instructor Solution B.** The instructor asks the student to leave the class since the student doesn't like how things are going.

❑ **Instructor Solution C.** The instructor asks the student to meet him in his office and confronts the student in private. During the meeting, the instructor asks the student why he is constantly criticizing the course and what exactly the student would like to see. The instructor makes accommodations where possible.

Problem Behavior #2

A class includes a group of four students who always sit in the back corner of the classroom and talk among themselves quietly. Sometimes the conversation is based on the topics being discussed in the course. At other times, the conversation is totally unrelated to the course. During the third class session of the course, the instructor is tired of the disruption.

❑ **Instructor Solution A.** The instructor asks the students to leave the class.

❑ **Instructor Solution B.** The instructor tactfully uses humor to embarrass the students into not talking and to make them aware that they are being disruptive.

❑ **Instructor Solution C.** The instructor moves to the back of the class near the group of students while lecturing, regularly calls on them by name to answer questions or make comments, and politely and directly asks them to stop talking.

Problem Behavior #3

An instructor has a student who is often 15 minutes late to a 2-hour class reportedly because of transportation problems. The student is very bright, performing very well in school, and comes into class very discreetly. Another student has complained that the instructor isn't fair because she allows the student to be late without consequences.

- ❑ **Instructor Solution A.** The instructor penalizes the student in line with the syllabus, which will lower the student's final grade from an A to a B if the behavior continues throughout the course.
- ❑ **Instructor Solution B.** The instructor locks the door so that the student cannot enter the class late.
- ❑ **Instructor Solution C.** The instructor makes an allowance for the student's specific situation and tells the complaining student that the same allowances would be made for her if her situation were similar.

Problem Behavior #4

An instructor has a student in class who obviously has difficulty learning the material. The student's grades are below a C, and the student says that he spends a great deal of time studying the information but just doesn't seem to be able to learn it.

- ❑ **Instructor Solution A.** The instructor suggests to the student that this career, and subsequent career choice, doesn't seem to fit him. Since this is the "weeder" course for the program, it is obvious that he should choose something else that he finds easier. He sends the student to his advisor to change majors or drop from school.
- ❑ **Instructor Solution B.** The instructor agrees that the course is difficult and requires a great deal of work. The instructor then tells the student that obviously the student isn't working hard enough or spending enough time on the course and assigns additional work to help the student learn the material.
- ❑ **Instructor Solution C.** The instructor agrees that the course is difficult and asks the student to see him during office hours. During the meeting, the instructor questions on how the student is studying the material, makes suggestions for different studying strategies, and makes an appointment for the next week to discuss the results of the new studying strategies.

Problem Behavior #5

An instructor has a student that must have surgery during the course and plans to be out for no more than two weeks of a 12-week session. The student is a B student, very motivated to finish the course successfully, and is worried that the two weeks will put her too far behind to catch up. There is also a major project due during that two-week period. The student still has two weeks left in the class before she will be out.

- ❑ **Instructor Solution A.** The instructor explains that the student will probably not be able to successfully make up the lecture material, and will fail the project, since it will not be turned in on time. She suggests that the student drop the course and take it next term when she doesn't have the health problem.
- ❑ **Instructor Solution B.** The instructor gives the student her lecture notes for the two-week period she will miss and delays the deadline for the project until the student returns. During the two weeks she is still in class, the instructor makes a few appointments with the student to try to explain any difficult concepts in the material she will

miss. When the student returns after the surgery, the instructor makes additional appointments with the student to ensure that she has caught up on missed information.

❑ **Instructor Solution C.** The instructor allows the student to remain in the class and encourages her to catch up on the missed information as quickly as possible, perhaps getting the notes from a friend in class. She also states that she will take the assignment, but will lower the grade by 10% since it will be late.

Problem Behavior #6

Describe a problem behavior or situation that you have recently experienced in your own course.

❑ **Instructor Solution A.** Describe an ineffective solution that you know some instructors might choose.

❑ **Instructor Solution B.** Describe a solution that you know some instructors might choose and that looks fair, but that does not help students meet their academic and career goals.

❑ **Instructor Solution C.** Describe an effective solution that will both assist students in meeting their academic and career goals as well as maintain the integrity of the course and institution.

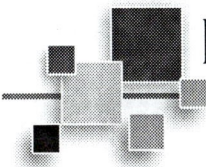

INSTRUCTOR IMPROVEMENT PLAN

Suggestions for Completing this Plan

1. Take the Premodule Assessment to determine your baseline knowledge of classroom management techniques.
2. Read the outline and note the objectives of the *Teacher Training Boot Camp* module. Doing so will provide you with background information that will help you better assess your skill level in these areas.
3. Compose a list of questions for which you would like to find answers or topics you wish to explore in this section.
4. Use the information obtained from suggestions one through three above to complete this plan.

AREAS OF STRENGTH

Based on the information gathered by completing the Premodule Assessment, reviewing the objectives and outline, and composing your list of questions and topics, list your strongest skills and knowledge in the areas discussed. These items should reflect things that you currently do in your classroom that you believe to be your strongest assets.

AREAS FOR DEVELOPMENT

Again, based on the information gathered by completing the recommended activities above, create a list of general areas in which you feel you could develop your ability to help students learn to learn. These should be general areas, such as "developing your presentation skills" or "understanding more about using learning theory in the classroom." These general areas will be used to develop specific goals.

GOAL SETTING

A format in table form for setting goals and identifying resources can be found on the following page. One plan should be completed for each long-term goal that you establish. When writing your goals, the following guidelines are suggested:

1. Goals should be realistic and achievable. Considering your other life commitments, time availability, and other aspects of your particular situation, set goals that you can realistically achieve and that will provide you with a sense of accomplishment.

2. Write goals that are understandable. Be clear and concise. Your goals should be clearly stated so when you review them in the future, you can plainly understand the direction in which you planned to head. Likewise, a supervisor or colleague should also be able to clearly understand your intention when reading your goals.

3. Your goals should be measurable. In other words, there should be a concrete, observable product or behavior at the completion of each goal. When this product or behavior is satisfactory, you will know your goal has been achieved. Write your goals to reflect behavioral outcomes that you or another individual can observe.

4. Break your goals into long-term and short-term components. The long-term goal reflects the final outcome that you wish to achieve. The short-term component outlines the smaller elements that you will complete en route to completing the long-term goal. Short-term goals are helpful in gauging your progress toward completing your larger objective.

5. Review and revise goals regularly. Evaluate your goals and your progress periodically and on a regular basis. Goals can certainly be revised and revamped as your needs suggest. The Instructor Improvement Plan format provides an option for revisiting and revising your goals. A change to a goal does not mean failure.

6. Brainstorm sources of information that will provide you with resources for completing your goal. Resources can take many forms, including print material, electronic and audiovisual media, professional organizations, and supervisors or mentors, to name a few. Establish a general idea of where you wish to find information and investigate your possibilities. You may be surprised at the additional resources that present themselves as you complete this process.

INSTRUCTOR IMPROVEMENT PLAN

Name: _____ Date Developed: _____

Long-Term Goal:					
SHORT-TERM GOALS	**METHOD AND RESOURCES FOR ACHIEVING GOAL**	**TARGET DATE FOR COMPLETION**	**DATE COMPLETED**	**OUTCOMES**	**REVISION/DATE**

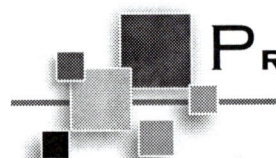

PROFESSIONAL DEVELOPMENT PORTFOLIO

PORTFOLIO ORGANIZATION SUGGESTIONS

I. Portfolio Part 1: Introduction

- Premodule Assessment*
- Initial Instructor Improvement Plan and Reflection*

II. Portfolio Part 2: Resource Development

(Include information that you print from the module or find in support of the learning activities.)

Section 1: An Overview of Instructor Responsibilities and Learning Theory
- Essential Workplace Skills Analysis (Include a list of ideas that result from the analysis of essential workplace skills including how you can support these skills in your classroom.)
- Student Population Exploration (Include a brief analysis of the student population you are teaching.)
- Learning and Instructional Theory Research (Include a detailed ongoing reference list for learning and instructional theory.)
- Bloom's Taxonomy (Include the Bloom's Taxonomy Word List.)
- Teaching Hands-on Skills (Include the Teaching Hands-on Skills Worksheet.)
- Learning Style Discovery (Include the references for learning style inventories and the Addressing Different Learning Styles Checklist.)

Section 2: Preparing to Teach and the First Days of Class
- Syllabus Development (Include the Course Syllabus Template.)
- First Day of Class Agenda (Include the Sample First Day Agenda.)
- Textbook Research (Include the Textbook Selection Checklist.)
- Equipment, Facilities, and Technology (Include the Equipment, Facilities, and Technology Worksheet.)
- Activity Development (Include the Activity Development Worksheet.)
- Ice-Breakers (Include a list of ice-breakers you can use for first-day introductions. Continue adding to this list as you find new ideas. Also include an evaluation of each activity as you try it with ideas for revision, if needed.)

Section 3: The Day-to-Day Classroom Environment
- Active Learning (Include the Idea List for Classroom Activities.)
- Critical-Thinking Research (Include a list of references for critical-thinking strategies and activities.)
- Instructor Attitudes (Include the Instructor Characteristics Rating Sheet.)

Section 4: Grading and Assessment
- Plagiarism Software Research (Include an ongoing list of plagiarism software with a brief synopsis and critique of each.)

- Electronic Exam Generator Software (Include an ongoing list of references for electronic exam generator software with a brief synopsis and critique of each.)
- Feedback (Include the Feedback Assessment Checklist.)

Section 5: Effective Classroom Management Strategies
- Attitude Assessment (Include the Instructor Attitude Rating Form.)
- Online Research for Advising Students (Include an ongoing list of references to assist in advising students.)

III. Portfolio Part 3: Practice and Development: Activities and Reflections

Section 1: An Overview of Instructor Responsibilities and Learning Theory
- Reflection Questions (Complete the reflection questions diligently and add them to the portfolio. Some of your responses to reflection questions will provide examples and feedback that will complement other portfolio artifacts.)
- Essential Workplace Skills Analysis (Include a list of ideas that result from the analysis of essential workplace skills, including how you can support these skills in your classroom.)
- Learning and Instructional Theory Research (Include a detailed and ongoing list of specific learning theories you investigate, including specific ways you could incorporate these theories into your teaching.)
- Learning Style Discovery (Include an analysis of your personal learning style and ways you might need to alter your natural teaching in order to address different learning styles in your classroom.)

Section 2: Preparing to Teach and the First Days of Class
- Reflection Questions (Complete the reflection questions diligently and add them to the portfolio. Some of your responses to reflection questions will provide examples and feedback that will complement other portfolio artifacts.)
- Syllabus Development (Include a detailed syllabus for one or two of the courses you teach.)
- First Day of Class Agenda (Include an agenda for the first day of class. Start with a list of first-day objectives and why these are important.)
- Textbook Research (Include an analysis of a textbook you have used for your course.)

Section 3: The Day-to-Day Classroom Environment
- Reflection Questions (Complete the reflection questions diligently and add them to the portfolio. Some of your responses to reflection questions will provide examples and feedback that will complement other portfolio artifacts.)
- Active Learning Assignment (Include a list of activities for your course as a demonstration of how you incorporate active learning into the class.)
- Keeping Students Engaged (Include an idea list resulting from your brainstorming session organized by topic area.)
- Critical-Thinking Research (Include a list of references for critical-thinking strategies and activities.)
- Instructor Attitudes (Include the results of your Instructor Characteristics Rating Sheet and a discussion of areas in which you can improve and an action plan for that improvement.)

Section 4: Grading and Assessment
- Reflection Questions (Complete the reflection questions diligently and add them to the portfolio. Some of your responses to reflection questions will provide examples and feedback that will complement other portfolio artifacts.)
- Grading Policies (Insert an example of your grading policies with a justification for each policy and how it helps students succeed in your course.)
- Course Assessment Brainstorming (Include an ongoing list of ways to assess your students organized by topic.)

Section 5: Effective Classroom Management Strategies
- Reflection Questions (Complete the reflection questions diligently and add them to the portfolio. Some of your responses to reflection questions will provide examples and feedback that will complement other portfolio artifacts.)
- Attitude Assessment (Include the results of your attitude assessment and an action plan for improvement. Also include the follow-up assessment after you have had sufficient time to implement your plan. Discuss the differences and set a new plan and time frame if needed.)
- Dealing with Problem Behavior (Include the results of your problem behavior discussion based on the Student Problem Behavior Worksheet.)

IV. Portfolio Part 4: Feedback

(Include information from your class evaluations and instructor observations.)

Section 1: An Overview of Instructor Responsibilities and Learning Theory
- Include feedback on how you meet instructor responsibilities.
- Include feedback on how you use learning theory in your teaching.

Section 2: Preparing to Teach and the First Days of Class
- Include feedback on your first-day-of-class activities and behaviors.

Section 3: The Day-to-Day Classroom Environment
- Include feedback on your presentation, discussion, questioning, and lecturing techniques.

Section 4: Grading and Assessment
- Include feedback on your grading policies and assessment effectiveness.

Section 5: Effective Classroom Management Strategies
- Include feedback on your skills in managing difficult situations in the classroom.

V. Portfolio Part 5: Reassessment

- Postmodule Assessment*
- Continuing Instructor Improvement Plan and Reflection* **

VI. Portfolio Part 6: Capstone

Section 1: An Overview of Instructor Responsibilities and Learning Theory
- Learning and Instruction Theory Description and Application List

Section 2: Preparing to Teach and the First Days of Class
- First-Day-of-Class Agenda

Section 3: The Day-to-Day Classroom Environment
- Active Learning Assignment Listing

Section 4: Grading and Assessment
- Grading Policy and Procedure Document

Section 5: Effective Classroom Management Strategies
- Behavior Management List

* Pull for Professional Development Documentation Portfolio

** Pull for Showcase Portfolio

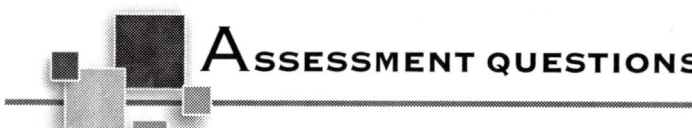

ASSESSMENT QUESTIONS

Section 1: An Overview of Instructor Responsibilities and Learning Theory

1. Discuss three responsibilities of an instructor and for each, provide ideas for meeting these responsibilities based on information from Section 1.

2. Discuss five characteristics of adult learners and for each characteristic listed, suggest two strategies for facilitating learning.

3. Section 1 described visual, auditory, and kinesthetic learners. Select an activity and describe how you would modify it to meet the needs of each type of learner.

4. Select a topic from one of your classes and for that topic, write a question or activity that reflects Bloom's cognitive levels of knowledge, comprehension, application, analysis, synthesis, and evaluation.

5. Select a topic and describe how you would teach it using the Cognitive Apprenticeship Model steps of model, coach, scaffold, articulate, reflect, and explore.

Section 2: Preparing to Teach and the First Days of Class

6. Discuss four considerations to make when reviewing a textbook prior to a course.

7. Discuss the importance of a well-organized syllabus and describe at least five elements that the syllabus should contain.

8. Describe four considerations when creating classroom activities and explain the importance of each.

9. Describe two alternatives to a traditional grade book.

10. Describe four strategies for maximizing success on the first day of class. Explain the goal of each strategy you select.

Section 3: The Day-to-Day Classroom Environment

11. Discuss the importance of establishing rapport with adult learners. List at least three types of information that contribute to establishing rapport, and explain why each is important in terms of adult learning.

12. Describe four components of using lecture effectively. For each, provide an example of how the component can be incorporated into your own classes.

13. Explain three characteristics of effective questioning in the classroom. Explain how each characteristic that you select enhances the questioning process.

14. Explain three benefits of discussion for students.

15. Select two approaches to conflict resolution. Explain when you would use each and give an example from the classroom.

16. List and describe the steps you would take in approaching conflict resolution with a student.

17. Explain the four components of active learning, and for each, give an example of an activity that could be used in your class.

Section 4: Grading and Assessment

18. Describe three purposes of assessment in the classroom.

19. Describe three appropriate goals for giving feedback to students.

20. Explain the steps of giving effective feedback.

21. Select three of Bloom's cognitive levels, and for each, describe an activity that assesses effectively at that level. Explain your rationale for selecting the activity according to Bloom's taxonomy.

22. Propose a grading process that is equitable and directed at minimizing grade-related complaints. Use at least four points from the module in your response.

23. Discuss three strategies for promoting academic honesty in the classroom.

Section 5: Effective Classroom Management Strategies

24. Select two of the reasons for low motivation in students, and for each, prescribe an approach that reflects what an instructor should do for the student. Explain two approaches that an instructor should *not* take with the student.

25. Describe a safe learning environment and suggest three strategies for creating one. Explain how a safe learning environment contributes to adult learners' success and motivation.

26. Select two problem behaviors that can be encountered in the classroom and that are described in the module. Describe each and suggest two approaches for addressing each behavior.

27. Summarize the importance of supporting the institution and provide two strategies for doing so.

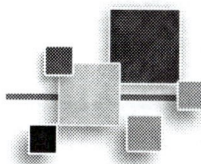

Assessment answer key

The following are references to the answers for the Assessment Questions for the Boot Camp Module. Information that serves as the basis for the answers in this section can be found in Sections 1–5. To make the information relevant to you, apply it thoughtfully to your individual situation.

Section 1: An Overview of Instructor Responsibilities and Learning Theory

1. Discuss three responsibilities of an instructor and for each, provide ideas for meeting these responsibilities based on information from Section 1.

   Answer should make reference to the Suggested General Guidelines: Responsibilities of Instructors section. The answer may also include any information from other parts of Section 1. Relationships of information to instructor responsibility should be thoroughly and clearly stated.

2. Discuss five characteristics of adult learners and for each characteristic listed, suggest two strategies for facilitating learning.

   Answer should make reference to the following:

   - Adult Learners in a Nutshell section; all subheadings
   - Bulleted points that suggest strategies for supporting the adult learner

3. Section 1 described visual, auditory, and kinesthetic learners. Select an activity and describe how you would modify it to meet the needs of each type of learner.

   Answer should make reference to the Selected Educational Theories for the Adult Learner section; Learning Styles subheading.

4. Select a topic from one of your classes and for that topic, write a question or activity that reflects Bloom's cognitive levels of knowledge, comprehension, application, analysis, synthesis, and evaluation.

   Answer should make reference to the Selected Educational Theories for the Adult Learner section; Bloom's Taxonomy subheading.

5. Select a topic and describe how you would teach it using the Cognitive Apprenticeship Model steps of model, coach, scaffold, articulate, reflect, and explore.

   Answer should make reference to the Selected Educational Theories for the Adult Learner section; The Cognitive Apprenticeship Model subheading.

Section 2: Preparing to Teach and the First Days of Class

6. Discuss four considerations to make when reviewing a textbook prior to a course.

   Answer should make reference to the following:

   - Textbook Selection and Review section
   - General Strategies for Textbook Selection and Review section

7. Discuss the importance of a well-organized syllabus and describe at least five elements that the syllabus should contain.

Answer should make reference to the following:

- Development of Course Materials section
- General Strategies for Developing the Syllabus section

8. Describe four considerations when creating classroom activities and explain the importance of each.

   Answer should make reference to the following:

   - Development of Course Materials section
   - General Strategies for Developing the Learning Activities section

9. Describe two alternatives to a traditional grade book.

   Answer should make reference to the Grade Book Organization section; Electronic Grade Books subheading.

10. Describe four strategies for maximizing success on the first day of class. Explain the goal of each strategy you select.

    Answer should make reference to the following:

    - The First Day of Class section
    - General Strategies for Having a Successful First Day section

Section 3: The Day-to-Day Classroom Environment

11. Discuss the importance of establishing rapport with adult learners. List at least three types of information that contribute to establishing rapport, and explain why each is important in terms of adult learning.

    Answer should make reference to the following:

    - Establish Rapport section
    - General Strategies for Establishing Rapport section (Understand Your Audience bullet)

12. Describe four components of using lecture effectively. For each, provide an example of how the component can be incorporated into your own classes.

    Answer should make reference to the following:

    - Be an Excellent Lecturer section
    - General Strategies for Using Lecture Effectively section

13. Explain three characteristics of effective questioning in the classroom. Explain how each characteristic that you select enhances the questioning process.

    Answer should make reference to the following:

    - Effective Questioning section
    - General Strategies for Effective Questioning section

14. Explain three benefits of discussion for students.

    Answer should make reference to the Facilitating Discussion section.

15. Select two approaches to conflict resolution. Explain when you would use each and give an example from the classroom.

    Answer should make reference to the Conflict Resolution section.

16. List and describe the steps you would take in approaching conflict resolution with a student.

    Answer should make reference to the following:

    - Conflict Resolution section
    - General Strategies for Resolving Conflict section

17. Explain the four components of active learning, and for each, give an example of an activity that could be used in your class.

    Answer should make reference to the Using Active Learning Techniques section.

Section 4: Grading and Assessment

18. Describe three purposes of assessment in the classroom.

    Answer should make reference to the following:

    - Suggested General Guidelines: Assessment and Evaluation of the Adult Learner section
    - General Strategies for Using Assessment section

19. Describe three appropriate goals for giving feedback to students.

    Answer should make reference to the Providing Effective Feedback section.

20. Explain the steps of giving effective feedback.

    Answer should make reference to the following:

    - Providing Effective Feedback section
    - General Strategies for Providing Feedback section

21. Select three of Bloom's cognitive levels, and for each, describe an activity that assesses effectively at that level. Explain your rationale for selecting the activity according to Bloom's taxonomy.

    Answer should make reference to the Building Assessment Tools section; all sub-headings related to Bloom.

22. Propose a grading process that is equitable and directed at minimizing grade-related complaints. Use at least four points from the module in your response.

    Answer should make reference to the following:

    - Grading Policies section
    - General Strategies for Establishing Equitable and Fair Grading Policies section
    - General Strategies for Reducing Grade-Related Complaints section

23. Discuss three strategies for promoting academic honesty in the classroom.

    Answer should make reference to the following:

    - Promoting Academic Integrity section
    - General Strategies for Promoting Academic Integrity section

Section 5: Effective Classroom Management Strategies

24. Select two of the reasons for low motivation in students, and for each, prescribe an approach that reflects what an instructor should do for the student. Explain two approaches that an instructor should *not* take with the student.

    Answer should make reference to the Student Motivation section (all subheadings, all bullets).

25. Describe a safe learning environment and suggest three strategies for creating one. Explain how a safe learning environment contributes to adult learners' success and motivation.

    Answer should make reference to the following:

    - Safe Learning Environments section
    - General Strategies for Creating Safe Learning Environments section

26. Select two problem behaviors that can be encountered in the classroom and that are described in the module. Describe each and suggest two approaches for addressing each behavior.

    Answer should make reference to the Problem Behaviors section (all subheadings, all bullets).

27. Summarize the importance of supporting the institution and provide two strategies for doing so.

    Answer should make reference to the following:

    - Supporting Your Institution section
    - General Strategies for Supporting the Institution section

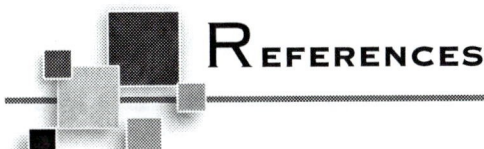
REFERENCES

Section 1: An Overview of Instructor Responsibilities and Learning Theory

Bloom, B. S. and Krathwohl, D. R. (1956). Handbook 1: Cognitive domain. *Taxonomy of educational objectives: The classification of educational goals by a committee of college and university examiners.* New York: Longman, Green.

Collins, A., Brown, J. S., & Newman, S. E. (1989). Cognitive apprenticeship: Teaching the craft of reading, writing and mathematics. In L. B. Resnick (Ed.), *Knowing, learning and instruction: Essays in honor of Robert Glaser* (pp. 453–494). Hillsdale, NJ: Erlbaum.

Kearsley, G. (1994–2004). *Explorations in learning & instruction: The theory into practice database.* Retrieved March 1, 2004, from http://tip.psychology.org/

Section 3: The Day-to-Day Classroom Environment

Cotton, K. (1988). Classroom questioning [Electronic version]. *School Improvement Research Series, Close-Up #5.* Northwest Regional Educational Laboratory. Retrieved March 15, 2004, from http://www.nwrel.org/scpd/sirs/3/cu5.html

Fink, L. D. (1999). *Active learning.* Retrieved March 15, 2004, from the University of Hawaii Honolulu Community College Web site: http://honolulu.hawaii.edu/intranet/committees/FacDevCom/guidebk/teachtip/active.htm

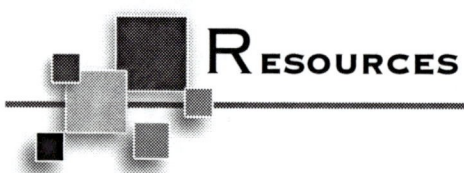

RESOURCES

ExamView. Retrieved November 21, 2004 from http://www.examview.com/. (ExamView is an easy-to-use electronic exam generator that utilizes textbook question pools and allows full custom question and exam development. From the home page, click on "Product Information" and "Features/Benefits.")

Kearsley, G. (1994–2004). *Explorations in learning & instruction: The theory into practice database.* Retrieved March 1, 2004, from http://tip.psychology.org/. (This is an excellent list of about fifty teaching and instructional theories created by Greg Kearsley in the online *Encyclopedia of Psychology.*)

U.S. Department of Education. *Accreditation in the United States.* Retrieved November 21, 2004, from http://www.ed.gov/. (This list links to both institutional and programmatic accrediting bodies. From the home page, click on the "Select a Topic" box. Click on "Accreditation.")

U.S. Department of Labor Bureau of Labor Statistics. Retrieved November 20, 2004, from http://www.bls.gov/. (This site can assist faculty in understanding the various career areas for students they teach. From the home page, click on "Occupations.")

Electronic Grade Book Examples

Class Action Grade Book. Retrieved November 21, 2004, from http://www.classactiongradebook.com. (From the home page, click on "Features" and "Frequently Asked Questions.")

Easy Grade Pro. Retrieved November 21, 2004, from http://www.easygradepro.com/. (From the home page, click on "About Easy Grade Pro" and "Features List.")

Grade Machine. Retrieved November 21, 2004, from http://www.mistycity.com. (From the home page, click on "Grade Machine.")

Grade Speed and Grade Speed Lite. Retrieved November 21, 2004, from http://www.gradespeed.net. (From the home page, click on "Products." Click on icons to learn more about the features.)

GradeQuick. Retrieved November 21, 2004, from http://www.jacksoncorp.com. (From the home page, click on "Learn About GradeQuick 9.")

Making the Grade. Retrieved November 21, 2004, from http://www.cri-mms.com. (From the home page, click on "Making the Grade" under the "Software Suite" contents list.)

Microsoft Office Templates: Education. Retrieved November 21, 2004, from http://www.microsoft.com. (Under "Popular Destinations," click on "Templates." Under "Browse Templates," click on "Education." Click on "For Teachers." Click on "Tests and Grades.")

ThinkWave. Retrieved November 21, 2004, from http://thinkwave.com. (From the home page, click on "Products," then click on "Learn More.")